STEMI VS. "FEMI"

A Real STEMI or a Fake STEMI

STEMI VS. "FEMI"

A Real STEMI or a Fake STEMI

HENRY K. SIU, MD
Attending Cardiologist
Interventional and General Cardiology
Mercer Bucks Cardiology; Jefferson Health

Thomas Jefferson University
Sidney Kimmel Medical College
Philadelphia, Pennsylvania

EDWARD H. SUH, MD
Contributing Editor
Emergency Medicine Attending
Assistant Professor of Medicine
Columbia University Medical Center
New York, New York

Assistant Medical Director
Emergency Department
New York-Presbyterian Allen Hospital
New York, New York

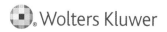

Philadelphia • Baltimore • New York • London
Buenos Aires • Hong Kong • Sydney • Tokyo

Senior Acquisitions Editor: Sharon R. Zinner
Development Editor: Ashley Fischer
Editorial Coordinator: Alexis Pozonsky
Editorial Assistant: Virginia Podgurski
Marketing Manager: Rachel Mante Leung
Production Project Manager: Marian Bellus
Design Coordinator: Joan Wendt
Prepress Vendor: Newgen Knowledge Works Pvt. Ltd., Chennai, India

9 8 7 6 5 4 3 2 1

Printed in China

9781496383136
Library of Congress Cataloging-in-Publication Data
available upon request

LWW.com

Dedication

Thank you to my family, in particular, my loving wife, Xiao, my two children, and my parents for their unwavering support.

Also, not to forget the friends, teachers, and patients who I have crossed paths with and have gotten me to this point.

Preface

 In modern healthcare, the art of medicine has met the push for established protocols: none more striking than the established plan for the rapid diagnosis and management of an ST-segment elevation myocardial infarction ("STEMI").

STEMI protocols have changed how we react to a common cardiac emergency for the better. However, they have also increased potential for poor judgment as rushed decisions without investigating complete medical history, as we are pressured to meet the 90-minute "door-to-balloon-time."

Not everything in medicine is cut and dry, or black and white. Although on paper the diagnosis of a STEMI is straightforward, in reality, it can be challenging.

ST elevation does not always equate to an acute coronary vessel occlusion. We are often faced with **mimics of STEMI,** which I will term "**FEMI,**" as in "**F**ake ST **E**levation **MI**."

The distinction between a STEMI and a "FEMI" is of utmost importance. A true STEMI is a medical emergency. Immediate care must be provided to the patient and the interventional cardiology service must be alerted with the goal of restoring blood flow to the heart as soon as possible. It is a US hospital quality-metric and an American College of Cardiology and American Heath Association (ACC/AHA) guideline recommendation to restore cardiac blood flow via percutaneous coronary intervention in 90 minutes on presentation ("door-to-balloon-time"). Given the acute nature of this disease, it is crucial to interpret the first electrocardiogram (ECG) in an expedited and accurate manner.

The ACC/AHA specifies that a 12-lead ECG should be **obtained and interpreted with a goal of within 10 minutes of arrival for patients presenting with chest discomfort or symptoms suspicious for acute coronary syndromes**. This gives intense pressure to quickly and accurately diagnose a STEMI (and to exclude a FEMI).

Unfortunately, distinguishing STEMI from FEMI can often be difficult. Not recognizing STEMI can lead to serious adverse outcomes for the patients. Yet, committing to the diagnosis on STEMI and not recognizing mimics can also have serious consequences. Moreover, even after recognizing a STEMI suspected from a coronary artery occlusion, sometimes the next best action is not rushing the patient off to the cardiac catheterization laboratory for a coronary angiogram/ intervention, which carries inherent risks of the invasive procedure as it can be of more harm than benefit to the patient. Finally, there are instances in which the distinction between STEMI and FEMI cannot be entirely made, and the decision to pursue an emergent coronary angiogram cannot be avoided. **One must remember that an ECG, like any other medical evaluation or diagnostic test, can be fraught with "false-positives" and "false-negatives"—so that in the end, a sound clinical decision needs to be made.**

This book focuses on addressing these nuanced situations, which will hopefully help acute-care providers hone their diagnostic ability to better tailor therapy when the clinical question of myocardial ischemia is raised.

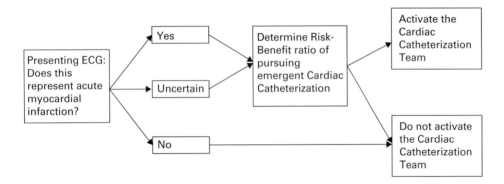

The above diagram illustrates the basic scheme for ECG interpretation and management in the acute setting, when the question of myocardial infarction is raised.

As an interventional cardiologist, I look forward to the opportunity to participate in the care of a patient with a STEMI. It always gives me a rush of adrenaline and each case teaches me something new. By the same token, I have been in cases where poor decisions led to unnecessary or even harmful activation of the catheterization laboratory team (at all hours of the day and night), whether it is the misinterpretation of the ECG itself or simply not realizing "The Big Picture" of the patient's underlying condition. Clearly, there is sometimes diagnostic uncertainty, and the consequence (both to the patient, and medico-legally, to the provider) in "missing" a STEMI diagnosis is not insignificant.

This is what inspired me to begin this collection of 100 cases.

For each case, I will provide the basic clinical vignette and one or more ECGs. I then ask you to answer two questions:

1. **Does the ECG demonstrate evidence of an acute myocardial infarction?**
2. **Would you activate the cardiac catheterization team as the next step in the patient's management?**

Henry K. Siu, MD

Guidelines: The ECG Diagnosis of STEMI

The following are the guidelines for the ECG diagnosis of STEMI on a standard 12-lead ECG[1]:

- In 2 or more contiguous leads, ST elevation at the J point ≥ 2 mm in leads V_2, and V_3 and ≥ 1 mm in all other leads.
- For men ≤ 40 years of age and older, ST elevation at the J point ≥ 2.5 mm in leads V_2 and V_3.
- For women, ST elevation at the J point ≥ 1.5 mm in leads V_2 and V_3.

For **posterior ECG leads**, ST elevation ≥ 0.5 mm is abnormal and suggestive of posterior ischemia in leads V_7, V_8, and V_9.

For **right-sided ECG leads**, ST elevation ≥ 0.5 mm in V_3R and V_4R is indicative of right ventricular (RV) infarction (except for males <30 years of age, for whom ≥ 1 mm is diagnostic).

Reference

1. Wagner GS, Macfarlane P, Wellens H, et al. AHA/ACCF/HRS recommendations for the standardization and interpretation of the electrocardiogram: part VI: acute ischemia/infarction. *J Am Coll Cardiol.* 2009;53(11):1003-1011 doi:10.1016/j.jacc.2008.12.016.

Contents

▸▸ CASE LIST

Case Number	STEMI vs. FEMI	Clinical Scenario	
1	STEMI	Mid-RCA	1
2	STEMI	Mid-LAD; serial ECGs	4
3	FEMI	Evolving ECG changes from recent MI	7
4	STEMI	LCx; posterior MI	10
5	FEMI	Critical aortic stenosis	15
6	FEMI	The automated ECG interpretation	17
7	STEMI	Proximal RCA; V4R showing RV involvement	20
8	STEMI	RCA, Wellens' T-wave syndrome	25
9	STEMI	Proximal RCA; are there two culprit lesions?	30
10	FEMI	Early repolarization	32

▶▶ CASE LIST

▶▶ **CASE LIST**

▶▶ CASE LIST

▶▶ CASE LIST

▶▶ CASE LIST

▶▶ STEMI CASE LIST BY CULPRIT VESSEL

Vessel	Case Number	Page Number
Left main	18, 35, _**72**_*	72, 133, 248
Left anterior descending (LAD)	2, 19, 24, 31, 37, 39, 46, 52, 54, 56, 59, 62, 67 (1st diagonal), _**70**_* (2nd diagonal), _**75**_*, 80, 84, 91	4, 75, 92, 118, 139, 145, 168, 189, 194, 199, 211, 219, 235, 242, 259, 273, 287, 310
Left circumflex (LCx) and Ramus Intermedius (RI)	4, 11, 14, 36, 49, 57, 61, 88	10, 38, 49, 136, 179, 203, 217, 296
Right coronary artery (RCA)	1, 7, 8, 9, 12, 20, 21, 23, 26, 27, _**28**_*, 30, 42, 43, 48, 50, 58, _**76**_*, 98, _**100**_*	1, 20, 25, 30, 44, 78, 81, 90, 100, 103, 106, 116, 154, 156, 174, 183, 209, 263, 335, 341
Myocardial ischemia with LBBB/ paced rhythm	11, 49, 57	38, 179, 203
Posterior MI	4, 36, 61, _**72**_*	10, 136, 217, 248

*See case explanation

CASE LIST BY CLINICAL SCENARIO

CASE LIST BY CLINICAL SCENARIO

Clinical Scenario	Case Number	Page Number
Hypercalemia	82	280
Hyperkalemia	44, 63, 78, 83, 88	159, 222, 268, 283, 296
Hypertensive emergency	66	232
Intracranial hemorrhage	41	152
Intraventricular conduction delay (IVCD)	17	68
Left bundle branch block (LBBB)	11, 33, 34, 49, 57	38, 126, 130, 179, 203
Left ventricular hypertrophy (LVH)	16, 17, 18, 19, 20, 45, 65, 66, 87, 99	60, 68, 72, 75, 78, 164, 229, 232, 294, 338
LV aneurysm	25, 71	97, 244
Multivessel coronary artery disease	9, 18, 21, 26, 29, 86	30, 72, 81, 100, 112, 292
Osborn wave/hypothermia	89	304
Pacemaker	49, 57, 83, 90, 95	179, 203, 283, 307, 329
Pericarditis	32, 55, 79, 92	122, 197, 270, 314
Pulmonary embolism	68, 93, 94	237, 317, 320
Retrograde P wave	81	277
Right bunble branch block (RBBB)	24, 27, 69	92, 103, 240
Serial ECG	2, 21, 31, 52, 56	4, 81, 118, 189, 199
Sgarbossa's criteria	11, 49, 57	38, 179, 203
Sinus pause	69	240

CASE LIST BY CLINICAL SCENARIO

Case 1

PRESENTATION

A 60-year-old male malpractice lawyer with active tobacco use and without known heart disease presents with acute shortness of breath and constant chest pain that radiates to his jaw. He also has mild nausea, and he says that he thinks these symptoms are from indigestion. He is very anxious and is asking many questions. The first troponin T was negative at <0.01 ng/mL (normal ≤ 0.01 ng/mL).

▸▸ **Presenting Electrocardiogram: Would You Activate the Cath Lab?**

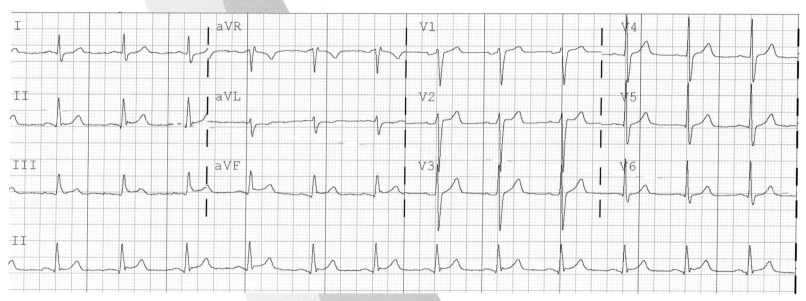

ECG 1.1

There is no prior electrocardiogram (ECG) available for comparison.

EXPLANATION

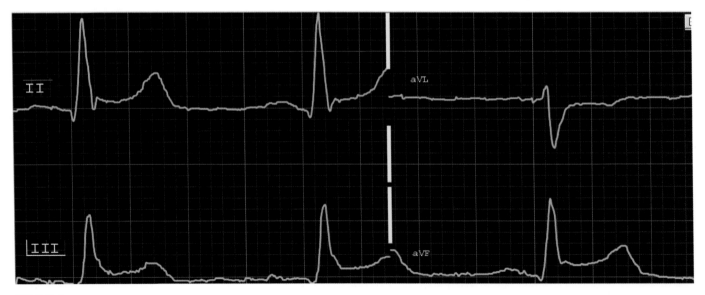

STEMI   The ECG demonstrates >1-mm elevation in the inferior leads (II, III, and aVF), and with reciprocal changes in lead aVL, consistent with acute inferior ST-elevation myocardial infarction (STEMI).

The following text gives a closer look at the inferior leads. The patient had a mid–right coronary artery (RCA) occlusion, and was treated with balloon angioplasty and stenting. At times, ECG changes even in acute vessel occlusion can be subtle, which gives rise to the following questions:

?

1. Why does the ST segment elevate in the setting of myocardial infarction?
2. And, why do some patients develop large "tombstone" ST elevations on ECG, while others have ECGs that barely meet the criteria for STEMI (as in this case)?

ECG 1.2

In brief, it is believed that the opening of sarcolemmal potassium-sensitive adenosine tri-phosphate (ATP) channels is the biomolecular basis for which ST elevations occur during acute myocardial ischemia.[1] In fact, genetic mutations or genetic polymorphisms of these cardiac sarco-lemmal channels, or even medications that could potentially modulate or affect the function of this channel (ie, sulfonylureas, which the patient was not taking) can cause patient-to-patient variation in the magnitude of ST-segment elevation during myocardial infarction.[1,2] There are conflicting data regarding the prognostic implication of ST-segment elevation magnitude in relation to the severity of myocardial injury and patient outcomes.[3-5]

As the first case in this book series, the relatively subtle ST elevations on this patient's presenting ECG should drive home the point that the diagnosis of an acute coronary occlusion can be difficult. Clinical judgment is essential to patient management in the emergent setting.

References

1. Li RA, Leppo M, Miki T, Seino S, Marbán E. Molecular basis of electrocardiographic ST-segment elevation. *Circ Res.* 2000;87(10):837-839.
2. Huizar JF, Gonzalez LA, Alderman J, Smith HS. Sulfonylureas attenuate electrocardiographic ST-segment elevation during an acute myocardial infarction in diabetics. *J Am Coll Cardiol.* 2003;42(6):1017-1021.
3. Aldrich HR, Wagner NB, Bostwick J, et al. Use of initial ST-segment deviation for prediction of final electrocardiographic size of acute myocardial infarcts. *Am J Cardiol.* 1988;61(10):749-753.
4. Clemmensen P, Grande P, Aldrich HR, Wagner GS. Evaluation of formulas for estimating the final size of acute myocardial infarcts from quantitative ST-segment elevation on the initial standard 12-lead ECG. *J Electrocardiol.* 1991;24(1):77-83.
5. Birnbaum Y, Criger DA, Wagner GS, et al. Prediction of the extent and severity of left ventricular dysfunction in anterior acute myocardial infarction by the admission electrocardiogram. *Am Heart J.* 2001;141(6):915-924.

Case 2

PRESENTATION

A 50-year-old male with known coronary artery disease (CAD) and previous stenting procedures presents after an episode of chest pain. His first electrocardiogram (ECG) was unrevealing for ischemia (see the following text). Initial cardiac enzymes were sent and were unremarkable. He subsequently became impatient in the emergency department, refused to stay for additional observation, and left against medical advice.

He returns within 4 hours via ambulance with a recurrent episode of chest pain along with radiation to the back.

▸▸ **Presenting Electrocardiogram: Would You Activate the Cath Lab?**

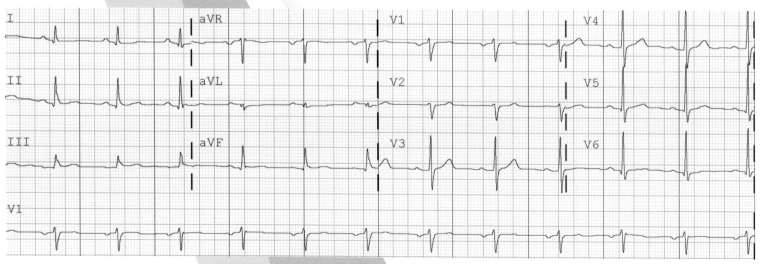

ECG 2.1

The patient subsequently leaves the emergency department against medical advice. The patient returns to the emergency department 4 hours later with recurrent symptoms (see ECG 2.2).

There is no prior ECG available for comparison.

▶▶ Repeat Electrocardiogram: Would You Activate the Cath Lab?

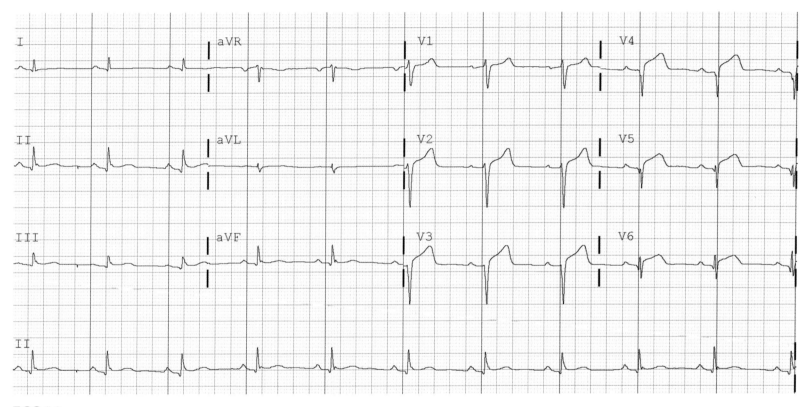

ECG 2.2

EXPLANATION

STEMI   The initial ECG was normal and was not suggestive of ischemia. The repeat ECG (when the patient was presented the second time to the emergency department) demonstrates new anteroseptal/anterior infarction with ST elevation in leads V_2 to V_6 and associated Q waves.

The patient was found to have a mid–left anterior descending coronary artery (LAD) 100% stenosis on catheterization when he returned to the hospital.

Cases like this are not uncommon, which underscores the need to carefully reevaluate the patients being managed for chest pain, even if the initial sets of diagnostics are unrevealing. This may include following through with serial cardiac serum biomarkers and ECGs.

From a pathophysiology standpoint, this patient likely had a plaque rupture prompting his initial visit to the emergency department, but the LAD had not thrombosed or have had enough acute platelet aggregation to cause flow-limiting vessel occlusion to create the ECG changes that demonstrate ischemia. Furthermore, the timing of his symptoms and presentation to the hospital was before the window of when serum troponin Ts were detectable, which is typically in the range of 3 to 4 hours after the onset of chest pain.

After the patient left the hospital, the ruptured plaque in the LAD (with the exposed tissue factor, pro-thrombotic milieu, and subsequently recruitment of activated platelets) had then progressed to vessel occlusion—leading to worsening symptoms and the patient's decision to return to the hospital.

Case 3

PRESENTATION

A 50-year-old male with multiple comorbidities including coronary artery disease (CAD), chronic obstructive pulmonary disease, and polysubstance abuse, presents with acute chest pain. He reports that he was treated for a "stent that had went down" 2 weeks ago at another hospital and that his current symptoms resemble that of his previous myocardial infarction presentation. The physicians are skeptical about his medication adherence to dual antiplatelet therapy and are therefore concerned about recurrent stent thrombosis.

▸▸ **Presenting Electrocardiogram: Would You Activate the Cath Lab?**

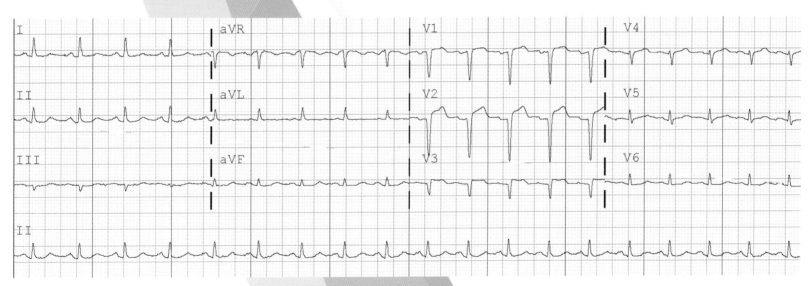

ECG 3.1

A prior electrocardiogram (ECG; from 1 month prior) is available for comparison (see ECG 3.2).

▶▶ Prior Electrocardiogram for Comparison

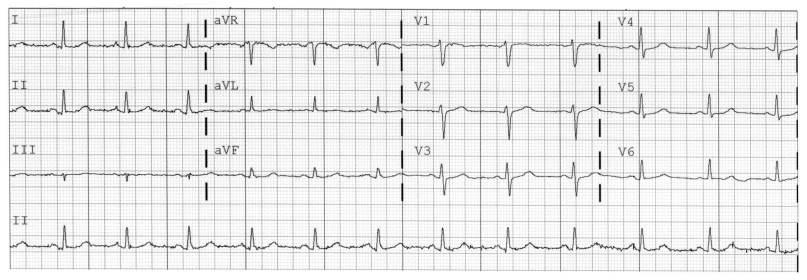

ECG 3.2

EXPLANATION

FEMI The ECG demonstrates sinus tachycardia, anterior/anteroseptal Q waves with ST elevations consistent with age-indeterminate infarction. These changes are new in comparison to previous ECG and are consistent with an ST-segment elevation myocardial infarction (STEMI).

Urgent catheterization, however, did not reveal new obstructive lesions, and the previous left anterior descending coronary artery (LAD) stent was patent.

In this case, the physicians were in a bind. The physicians did not have access to the patient's "**new baseline**" ECG after the recent hospitalization at another institution. The patient had been hospitalized for acute LAD stent thrombosis. After that ischemic event, his ECG had developed the persistent/evolving anterior Q waves with ST-T segment changes that were seen on his presenting ECG.

Not having access to previous available medical records in an emergent situation is not uncommon. One should be certain that the risk/benefits and alternative measures have been assessed before proceeding with emergent coronary angiogram in these scenarios, as additional information may dramatically change the risk–benefit ratio and necessity of proceeding with emergent coronary catheterization.

Case 4

PRESENTATION

A 54-year-old female with coronary artery disease (CAD) status post single-vessel coronary artery bypass graft (CABG; left internal mammary artery [LIMA] to left anterior descending coronary artery [LAD]), and a family history of premature CAD, presents with worsening chest pain and dyspnea over the past 2 days. She reports radiation of pain to the jaw, and that this is similar to the pain she had during her previous myocardial infarction.

▶▶ **Presenting Electrocardiogram: Would You Activate the Cath Lab?**

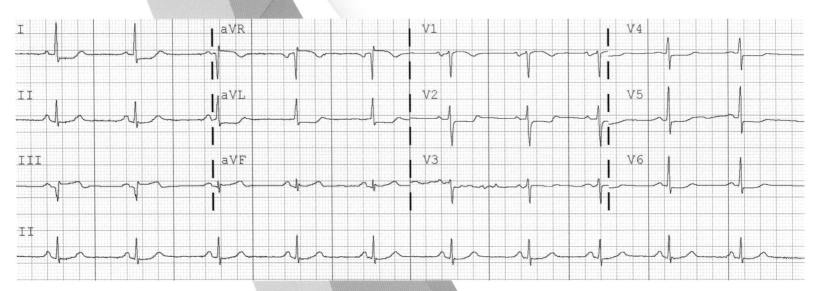

ECG 4.1

There is no prior electrocardiogram (ECG) available for comparison.

EXPLANATION

STEMI The ECG demonstrates ST depressions in V_1-V_3, a tall R wave in V_1 to V_3, with upright T wave in V_1 to V_3; this is consistent with an isolated posterior myocardial infarction. There is a 1-mm ST elevation in lead III, but it is in an isolated lead.

The patient had a culprit 99% stenosis in the mid–left circumflex coronary artery (LCx; after an OM1 branch) with significantly reduced flow. LCx ST-segment elevation myocardial infarctions (STEMIs) are notorious for being electrographically silent; this is due to the position of standard ECG leads and the anatomic position of the territory supplied by the LCx (often posterior). This is a scenario where a posterior lead ECG can be performed to confirm the diagnosis.

In this case, posterior leads (V_7, V_8, and V_9) may demonstrate ST elevation, suggestion of infarction in the infero-posterior territory supplied by the LCx artery. Of note, only ≥0.5 mm of ST elevation is required in leads V_7, V_8, and V_9 to be considered positive for acute ischemia/injury.[1]

▶▶ Placement of Posterior Electrocardiogram Leads[1]

Leads V_1, V_2, and V_3 are unchanged. Leads V_7, V_8, and V_9 take the place of V_4, V_5, and V_6, respectively, at the same horizontal level
Lead V_7 is at the posterior midaxillary line or in-between location of V_6 and V_8
Lead V_8 is at the mid-scapular line
Lead V_9 is left paraspinal
Note: ST elevation ≥0.5 mm is abnormal and suggestive of posterior ischemia in leads V_7, V_8, and V_9 (Figure 4.1 and ECGs 4.5 and 4.6).

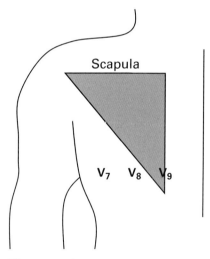

Scapula

V_7 V_8 V_9

Figure 4.1

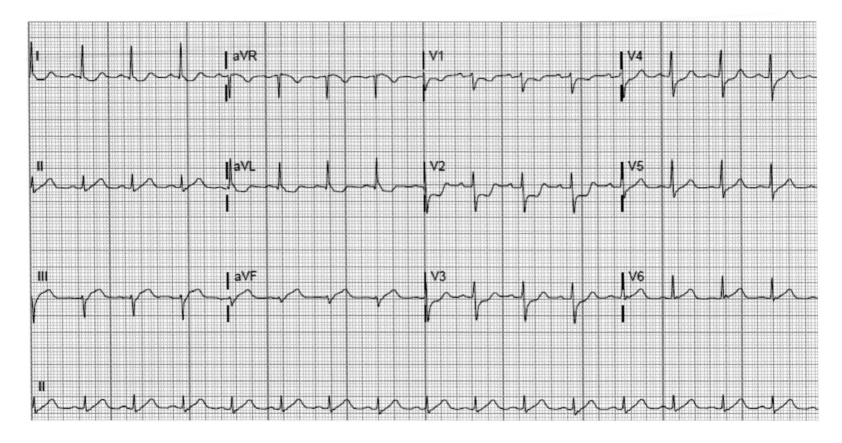

ECG 4.2

ECGs 4.2 is of a patient with a proximal LCx STEMI (infero-posterior infarction) that was confirmed by correctly utilizing the posterior leads; see ECGs 4.3.

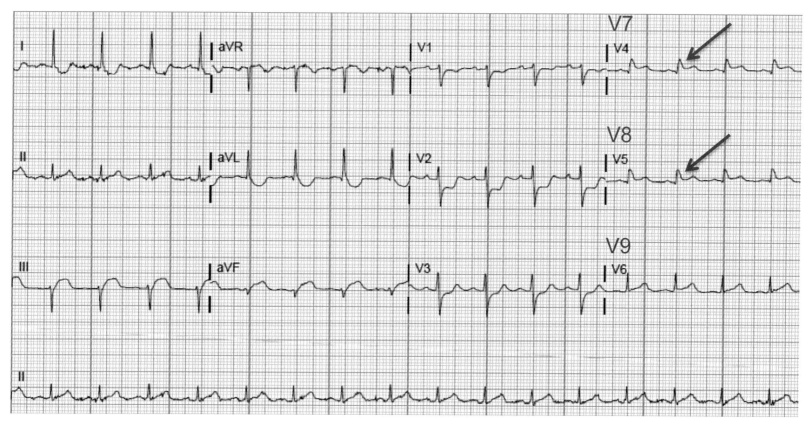

ECG 4.3

ECGs 4.3 is from the same patient scenario as ECGs 4.2. Note the >0.5-mm ST elevation in posterior leads (V_7 and V_8)—suggestive of posterior infarction extension, which is often difficult to realize with the standard 12 lead ECG.

Reference

1. Wagner GS, Macfarlane P, Wellens H, et al. AHA/ACCF/HRS recommendations for the standardization and interpretation of the electrocardiogram: part VI: acute ischemia/infarction: a scientific statement from the American Heart Association Electrocardiography and Arrhythmias Committee, Council on Clinical Cardiology; the American College of Cardiology Foundation; and the Heart Rhythm Society. Endorsed by the International Society for Computerized Electrocardiology. *J Am Coll Cardiol*. 2009;53(11):1003-1011. doi:10.1016/j.jacc.2008.12.016.

Case 5

PRESENTATION

A 77-year-old female with hypertension had an episode of syncope while walking on a busy street. Bystanders called 911. She did not reveal much about medical history on the way because she was slowly regaining her consciousness en route to the hospital.

In the emergency department, she is alert and oriented and seems to have a normal mental status. She denies active chest pain or shortness of breath.

▸▸ **Presenting Electrocardiogram: Would You Activate the Cath Lab?**

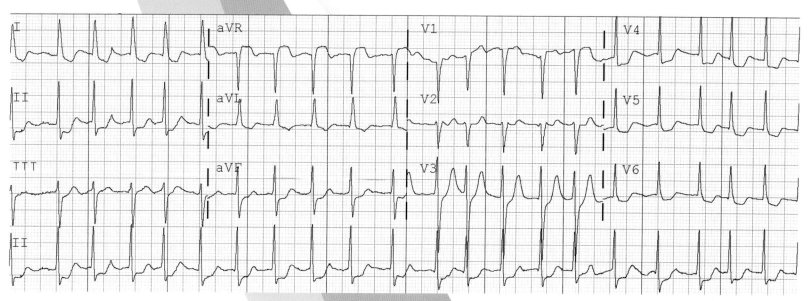

ECG 5.1

There is no prior electrocardiogram (ECG) available for comparison.

EXPLANATION

FEMI There are clear diffuse ST-T changes consistent with significant myocardial ischemia. Per guidelines, ST depression ≥1 mm on 8 or more leads coupled with ST-segment elevation in aVR and/or V_1, is suggestive of multivessel disease or left main disease.[1] However, in this case, the cause for the marked ST-T changes was not from acute coronary artery disease (CAD).

The cardiac catheterization team was emergently notified. The patient revealed she had untreated critical aortic stenosis. The patient had another syncopal episode while in the emergency department, which prompted an emergent balloon aortic valvuloplasty.

Without a doubt, the presenting ECG was indeed "high risk" by virtue of the ST depressions in multiple leads and elevation in aVR; coronary ischemia must be considered. Coronary angiography prior to the valvuloplasty revealed nonobstructiveCAD, and therefore, the ECG was consistent with major subendocardial ischemia, in the setting of atrial fibrillation with rapid ventricular response and critical aortic stenosis.

Emergent balloon aortic valvuloplasty was performed. Prior to the valvuloplasty, acute high-grade CAD was ruled out on catheterization. **Differential diagnoses of subendocardial ischemia include not only acute coronary syndromes, but also tachyarrhythmias, valvular disease, severe sepsis, or anemia with underlying severe CAD, and other causes of poor perfusion.**

The balloon (red arrow) dilates the stenotic aortic valve to allow for improved cardiac output (Figure 5.1).

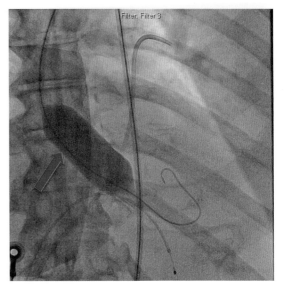

Figure 5.1

Reference

1. Wagner GS, Macfarlane P, Wellens H, et al. AHA/ACCF/HRS recommendations for the standardization and interpretation of the electrocardiogram: part VI: acute ischemia/infarction: a scientific statement from the American Heart Association Electrocardiography and Arrhythmias Committee, Council on Clinical Cardiology; the American College of Cardiology Foundation; and the Heart Rhythm Society. Endorsed by the International Society for Computerized Electrocardiology. *J Am Coll Cardiol.* 2009;53(11):1003-1011. doi:10.1016/j.jacc.2008.12.016.

Case 6

PRESENTATION

A 60-year-old male with a history of former tobacco use and hypertension presents to the primary care physician with symptoms of chest pain. It had been intermittent, substernal, and occurs infrequently with exertion. At the office visit, the patient's blood pressure was "slightly low," and the physician was worried about the possibility of a ST-segment elevation myocardial infarction (STEMI)-based on an electrocardiogram (ECG) obtained in the office.

The patient was sent by ambulance to the emergency department.

▶▶ **Presenting Electrocardiogram: Would You Activate the Cath Lab?**

Vent rate   69 bpm
PR interval   198 ms
QRS duration   85 ms
QT/QTc   411/441 ms
P-R-T axis 38 –25 34

Sinus rhythm
Borderline left axis deviation
Posterior infarct, acute (LCx)
Lateral infarct, old

– ABNORMAL ECG –

>>>> Acute MI <<<<

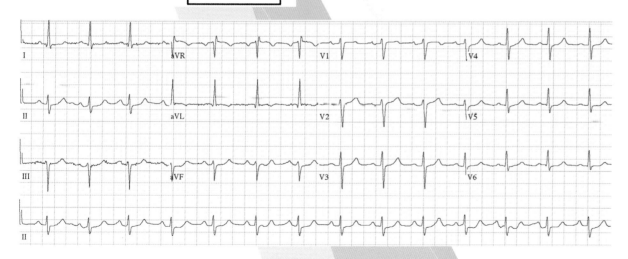

ECG 6.1

There is no prior ECG available for comparison, a repeat ECG was performed (see ECG 6.2).

▶▶ Repeat Electrocardiogram: Would You Activate the Cath Lab?

Vent rate	77 bpm
PR interval	221 ms
QRS duration	82 ms
QT/QTc	385/436 ms
P-R-T axis	41 −30 34

Sinus rhythm
Atrial premature complexes
Prolonged PR interval
Left atrial enlargement
Anteroseptal infarct, possibly acute
Inferolateral injury pattern
Prolonged QT
** ** ACUTE MI ** **
Abnormal ECG

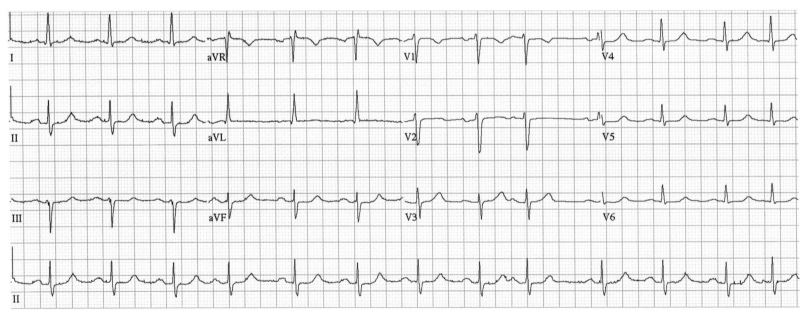

ECG 6.2

EXPLANATION

FEMI   Both the initial ECG at the primary care physician's office and in the emergency department are not consistent with an acute myocardial infarction. The automated ECG interpretation was registering ("over-reading") the nondiagnostic ST changes as acute ischemia.

Automated ECG interpretation is often quite accurate. **However, it is not yet as accurate as physician interpretation and should never replace clinical judgment. The automatic ECG interpretation should not be allowed to unduly influence your decision making.**

Cardiology consultation was called, but after review of the case, an urgent cardiac catheterization was aborted. This patient's cardiac biomarkers were negative, and he subsequently had a stress test that was negative for coronary ischemia.

Case 7

PRESENTATION

A 66-year-old male with a history of hypertension, but without known cardiac disease, presents with mid-scapular back pain and left-sided chest pain that awoke him from sleep.

In the emergency department, he is noted to be diaphoretic, bradycardic with heart rate 40 beats per minute (bpm) and hypotensive with systolic blood pressure in the 70s.

▶▶ **Presenting Electrocardiogram: Would You Activate the Cath Lab?**

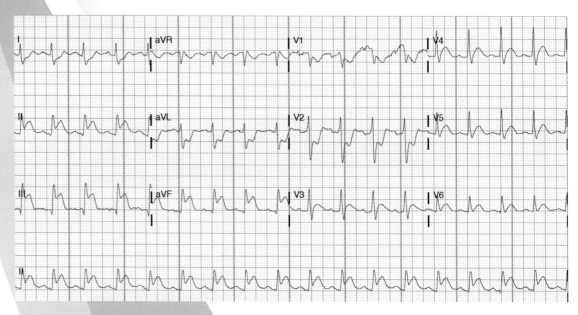

ECG 7.1

There is no prior electrocardiogram (ECG) available for comparison; a "right-sided" ECG was performed (see ECG 7.2).

▶▶ *"Right-Sided" Electrocardiogram*: Would You Activate the Cath Lab?

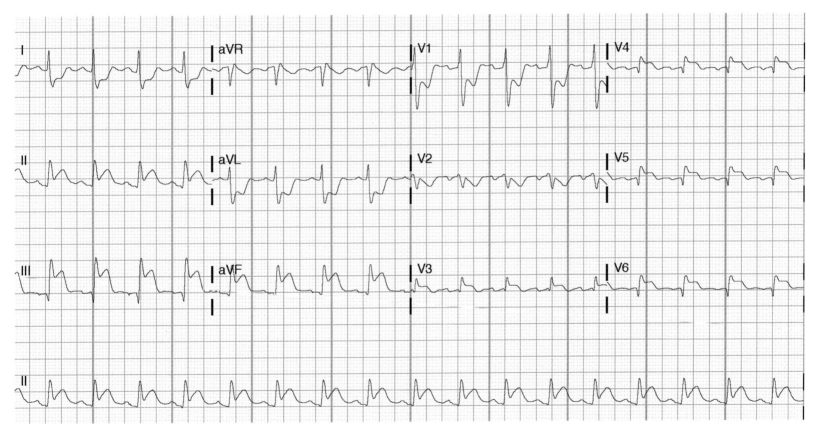

ECG 7.2

EXPLANATION

STEMI   The ECG demonstrates inferior lead ST elevations (II, III, and aVF) as well as ST depressions in leads V_1 to V_3, consistent with an inferior wall myocardial infarction (MI) with posterior extension (ECG 7.2). Right-sided leads demonstrate a right ventricular (RV) infarction.

Cardiac catheterization revealed an acute proximal right coronary artery (RCA) occlusion. The patient had prolonged hypotension and shock even after prompt revascularization of the RCA, but eventually recovered well with after and a period of inotropic support.

It is believed that 30% to 50% of patients with inferior–posterior wall MI will have RV infarction. Right-sided ECG will demonstrate RV involvement; ST elevation ≥0.5 mm in V_3R and V_4R is considered indicative of RV infarction (except for males <30 years of age, for whom ≥1 mm is diagnostic).[1,2] ST elevation in lead "V_4R" carries an 88% sensitivity and 78% specificity of detecting concurrent RV infarction in setting of inferior wall MI. Furthermore, RV infarction detected by this method is highly associated with increased morbidity and in-hospital mortality.[3] Familiarity with performing the right-sided ECGs may help identify a higher risk cohort of inferior wall MI patients (see Figure 7.1).

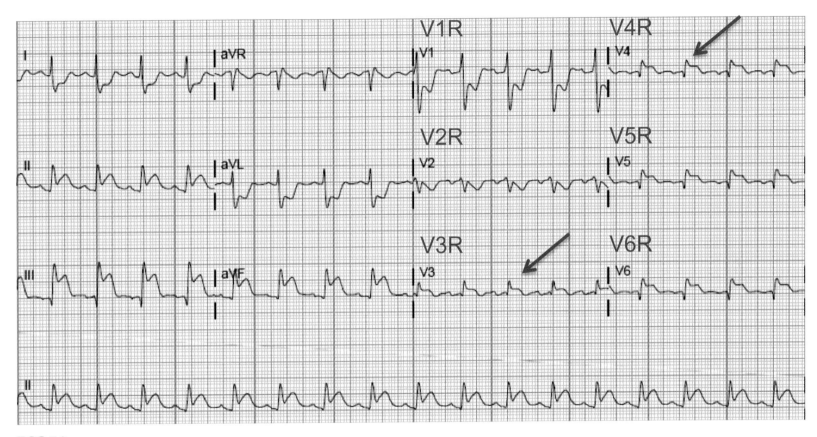

ECG 7.3

"Right-sided" ECG demonstrating RV infarction in setting of an inferior MI with ST elevation in lead V_4R (*red arrow*). ST elevation ≥0.5 mm in V_3R and V_4R is indicative of RV infarction (except for males <30 years of age, for whom ≥1 mm is diagnostic).

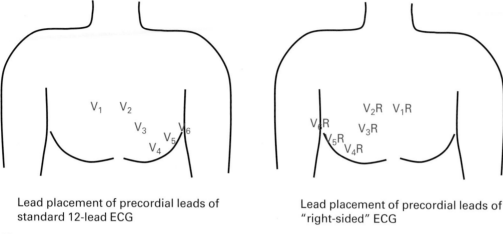

Lead placement of precordial leads of standard 12-lead ECG

Lead placement of precordial leads of "right-sided" ECG

Figure 7.1

References

1. Haji SA, Movahed A. Right ventricular infarction–diagnosis and treatment. *Clin Cardiol.* 2000;23(7):473-482.
2. Wagner GS, Macfarlane P, Wellens H, et al.; American Heart Association Electrocardiography and Arrhythmias Committee, Council on Clinical Cardiology; American College of Cardiology Foundation; Heart Rhythm Society. AHA/ACCF/HRS recommendations for the standardization and interpretation of the electrocardiogram: part VI: acute ischemia/infarction: a scientific statement from the American Heart Association Electrocardiography and Arrhythmias Committee, Council on Clinical Cardiology; the American College of Cardiology Foundation; and the Heart Rhythm Society. Endorsed by the International Society for Computerized Electrocardiology. *J Am Coll Cardiol.* 2009;53(11):1003-1011.
3. Zehender M, Kasper W, Kauder E, et al. Right ventricular infarction as an independent predictor of prognosis after acute inferior myocardial infarction. *N Engl J Med.* 1993;328(14):981-988.

Case 8

PRESENTATION

A 55-year-old female with hypertension, active tobacco smoking, and a history of esophageal surgeries for achalasia presents with chest pain with radiation to the jaw.

▸▸ **Presenting Electrocardiogram: Would You Activate the Cath Lab?**

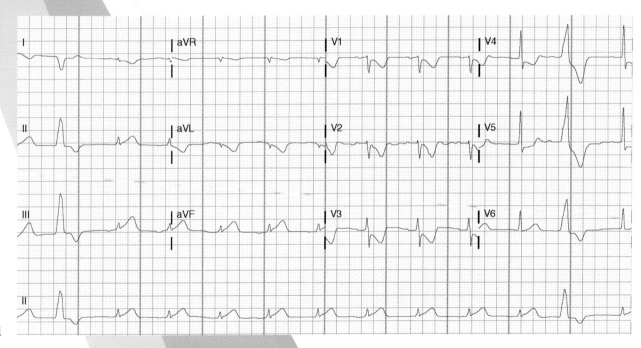

ECG 8.1

A prior electrocardiogram (ECG) is available for comparison (see ECG 8.2).

▶▶ Prior Electrocardiogram for Comparison

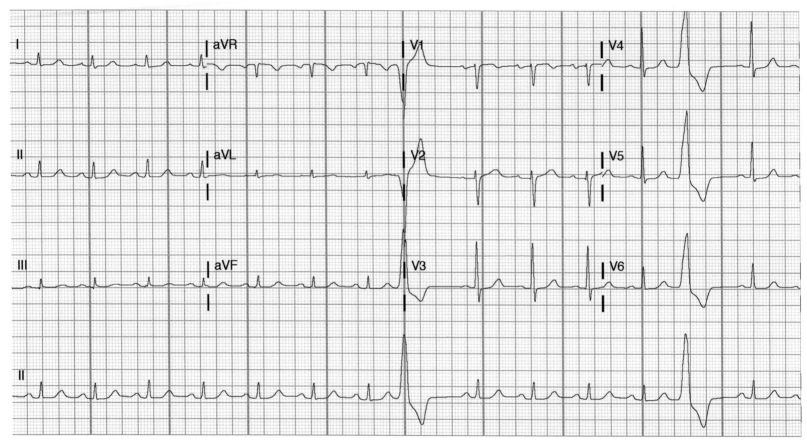

ECG 8.2

EXPLANATION

 STEMI   The ECG demonstrates inferior ST elevation with posterior extension; premature ventricular contractions are noted.

In this case, the acute myocardial infarction (MI) was not initially recognized because the physician was focused on the anterior T-wave inversions and was concerned for a Wellens' T-wave syndrome. Unfortunately, the inferior ST elevations were missed. Thirty minutes after the presenting ECG, the patient developed a ventricular fibrillation arrest in the emergency department, likely triggered by underlying acute ischemia.

"Wellens' T waves" is a pattern of deeply inverted or biphasic T waves in the anterior leads (V_2 and V_3), which have been considered highly specific for high-grade left anterior descending coronary artery (LAD) disease.[1] Sensitivity and specificity for significant stenosis of the LAD artery were found to be 69% and 89%, respectively, with a positive predictive value of 86%.[2] **Although the presenting ECG has dramatic anterior T-wave abnormalities, this was a manifestation of the posterior extension of the acute inferior wall ST-elevation MI.** It is important to carefully review the entire ECG and not focus only on obvious abnormalities.

▶▶ Wellens' T Wave: Example 1

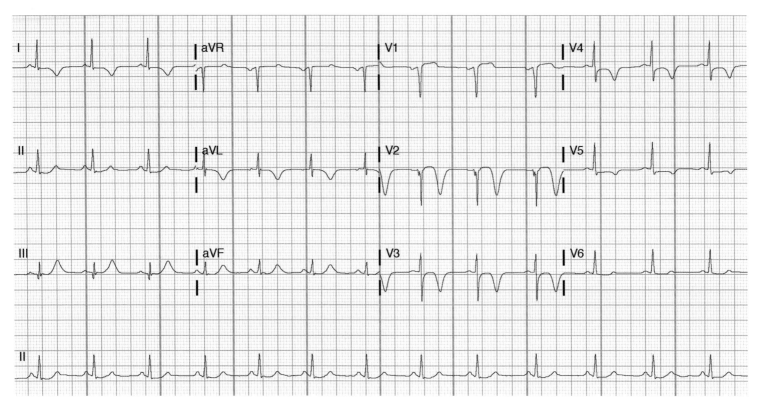

ECG 8.3

This is an ECG of a patient who presented with unstable angina. The ECG demonstrates deep biphasic T-wave inversions in the anterior leads. Although the ECG does not meet ST-segment elevation myocardial infarction (STEMI) criteria, the patient was triaged promptly for an urgent catheterization, which revealed the suspected critical proximal LAD stenosis.

▸▸ **Wellens' T Wave: Example 2**

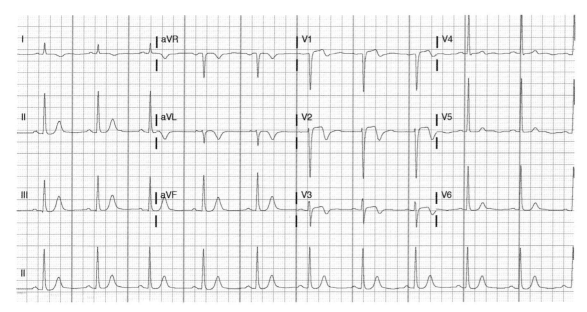

ECG 8.4

Similar to the previous example, this patient's ECG demonstrates deep biphasic T-wave inversions in the anterior leads consistent with Wellens' T waves. Cardiac catheterization revealed an unstable proximal LAD lesion and was treated with angioplasty and stenting.

References

1. de Zwaan C, Bär FW, Wellens HJ. Characteristic electrocardiographic pattern indicating a critical stenosis high in left anterior descending coronary artery in patients admitted because of impending myocardial infarction. *Am Heart J.* 1982;103(4 pt 2):730-736.
2. Haines DE, Raabe DS, Gundel WD, Wackers FJ. Anatomic and prognostic significance of new T-wave inversion in unstable angina. *Am J Cardiol.* 1983;52(1):14-18.

Case 9

PRESENTATION

A 52-year-old male without known medical history was witnessed collapsing on stress, apparently on the way to work. Bystanders reported that he appeared to be having chest pain prior to the loss of consciousness. Emergency medical services were called to the scene where advanced cardiovascular life support (ACLS) measures were initiated, including chest compressions and intravenous (IV) epinephrine. He was found to be in ventricular fibrillation and was defibrillated, which resulted in return of spontaneous circulation. He was brought to the emergency department after restoration of spontaneous circulation.

▸▸ **Presenting Electrocardiogram: Would You Activate the Cath Lab?**

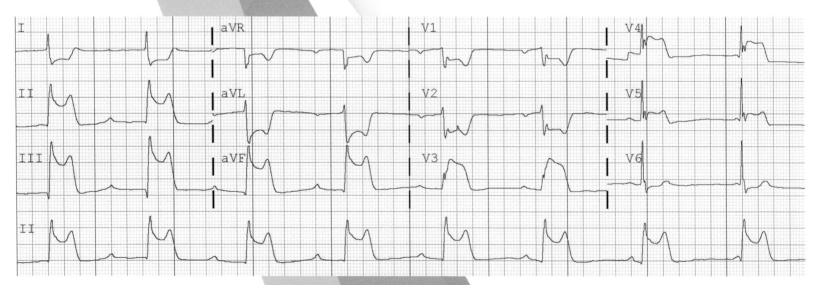

ECG 9.1

There is no prior electrocardiogram (ECG) available for comparison.

EXPLANATION

STEMI   The presenting ECG is rather interesting: Underlying complete heart block with ST elevations in the inferior and anterior leads. The patient's cardiac arrest with ventricular fibrillation was likely due to acute myocardial infarction (MI).

Catheterization revealed 100% stenosis of a dominant proximal right coronary artery (RCA) as the culprit lesion and was treated with angioplasty and stenting. This case is an example of clear ST elevations noted in a post–cardiac arrest ECG, and cardiac catheterization is warranted.

The question then becomes: *Why were there ST elevations in leads V_3, V_4, and V_5 (was there concomitant acute left anterior descending coronary artery [LAD] disease as well)?*

It turns out the patient did not have acute disease or high-grade obstructive lesions in the LAD. The anterior ST elevations may have been a result of global myocardial hypoxia from the cardiac arrest and vasoconstriction with IV epinephrine administered during the resuscitation.

Culprit lesion in the proximal RCA (*red arrow*), treated with balloon angioplasty and stenting. Notice the temporary pacemaker wire (*blue arrow*) for the complete heart block in setting of acute inferior MI (Figures 9.1 to 9.3).

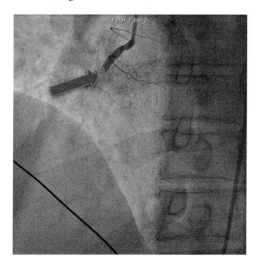

Figure 9.1

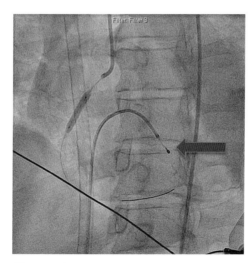

Figure 9.2

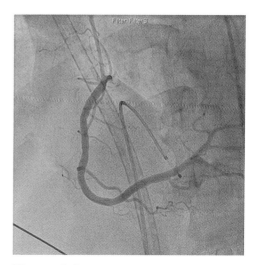

Figure 9.3

Case 10

PRESENTATION

A 52-year-old male without significant past medical history presents with shortness of breath, sore throat, fatigue, and cough. He also complains of mild exertional chest tightness and feels a lump in the throat.

▸▸ **Presenting Electrocardiogram: Would You Activate the Cath Lab?**

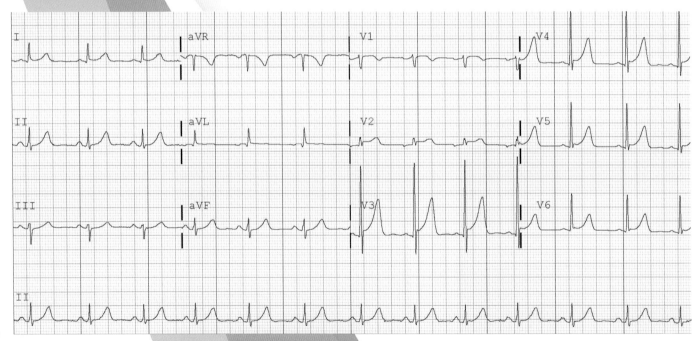

ECG 10.1

There is no prior electrocardiogram (ECG) available for comparison.

EXPLANATION

FEMI   The ECG demonstrates prominent 2-mm ST elevations in leads V$_3$ to V$_4$, and 1-mm elevation in lead V$_5$, which is indeed suspicious for anterior ischemia.

An urgent catheterization was performed and revealed normal coronaries despite the abnormal ST changes. In retrospect, the ECG is demonstrating a pattern of early repolarization.

Differentiating the ST changes of "benign" early repolarization from acute myocardial ischemia can be difficult but important. In general, 3 features favor the diagnosis of early repolarization over ST-segment elevation myocardial infarction (STEMI).

1. Concave ST—the "smiley" face.
2. Lack of reciprocal changes—ST depressions on leads without ST elevations.
3. Presence of QRS slurring/notching—patterns that require "pattern recognition."

The presenting ECG demonstrates concave ST, lack of reciprocal changes, and J-point elevation without QRS "slurring or notching" (Figure 10.1).

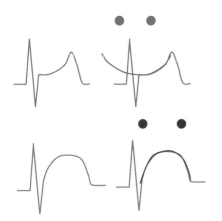

In the appropriate context, concave ST segment elevation can be described as a "smiley face" (green), which is often benign and favors the diagnosis of early repolarization.

On the contrary, when the ST segment is nonconcave or in the shape of an "unhappy face" (red), it is suspicious for myocardial ischemia.

Figure 10.1

Several early repolarization patterns exist, and these ST changes are not reflective of myocardial ischemia.[1] Recognizing the QRS "slurring" and "notching" patterns can be helpful in determining the presence of early repolarization (Figure 10.2).

The ECG definitions of early repolarization have not been standardized and even the cause of the ST-J segment deflections is still being debated (some evidence suggests these ST-J deflections are more accurately described as late depolarizations).[2] A consensus paper was published in 2015 in hopes of unifying the reporting for future research on this topic matter.[1] Utilizing the methodology from MacFarlane et al, the ST changes in leads V_2 to V_6 on the presenting ECG can be described as elevated J-point without ST slurring or notching.

The study of the early repolarization pattern has intensified since the landmark paper by Haïssaguerre et al[3] in 2008 suggested the presence of early repolarization may not truly be a "benign" finding. Their findings revealed an increased risk of idiopathic ventricular fibrillation that caused syncope and sudden cardiac death in patients younger than 60 years of age who had early repolarization pattern in the inferior and/or lateral leads on resting ECG.[3]

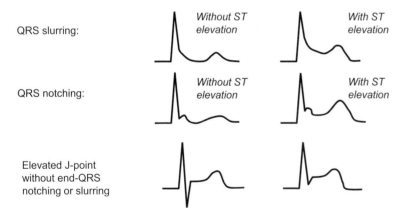

Figure 10.2

Adapted from MacFarlane et al.[1]

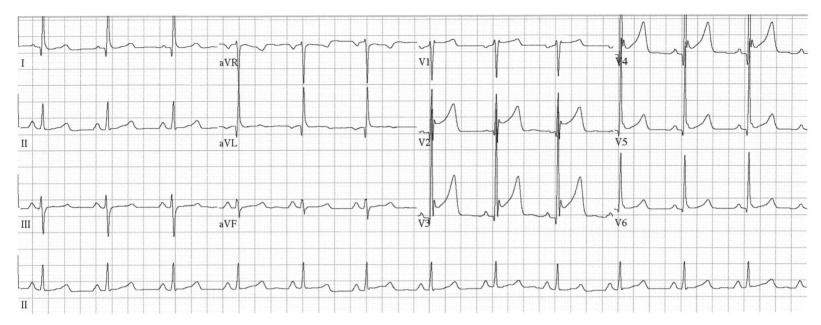

ECG 10.2

This is an example of early repolarization demonstrating "QRS notching" with ST elevations (leads V_2 through V_5), and "QRS slurring" without ST elevations in leads I and V_6. The presence of ST concavity and lack of reciprocal changes further supports early repolarization and not myocardial infarction.

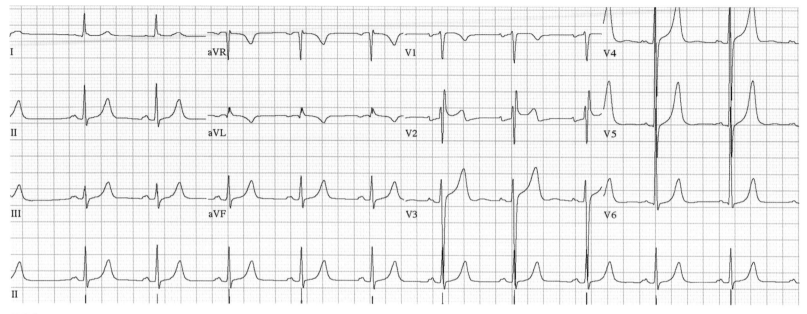

ECG 10.3

This patient's ECG demonstrates ST concavity ("smiley face" STs in lead V_2), no reciprocal changes, and QRS slurring with ST elevation in lead V_2, along with J-point elevation without end-QRS notching or slurring in V_3 and V_4. This is an example of early repolarization.

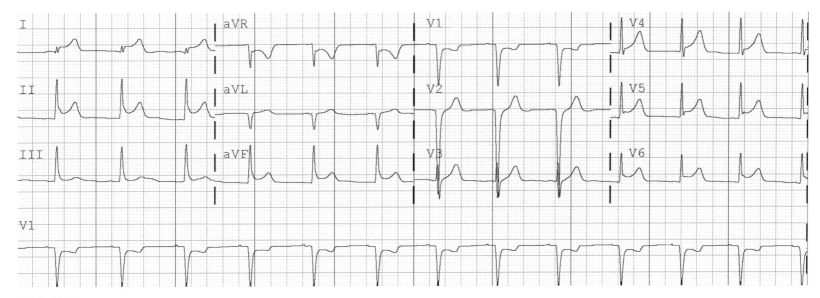

ECG 10.4

This is an ECG of a 35-year-old patient with ST elevations in the inferior and lateral leads. However, the ST elevations are not reflective of infarction. There are concave ST elevations ("smiley face" ST in leads with ST elevation), without reciprocal changes. This patient had normal coronaries on coronary angiogram and a structurally normal heart on echocardiogram. Studies suggest a higher than general risk for fatal ventricular arrhythmias when early repolarization pattern is seen on these leads.[3]

References

1. Macfarlane PW, Antzelevitch C, Haissaguerre M, et al. The early repolarization pattern: a consensus paper. *J Am Coll Cardiol.* 2015;66(4):470-477.
2. Spodick DH. Early repolarization: an underinvestigated misnomer. *Clin Cardiol.* 1997;20(11):913-914.
3. Haïssaguerre M, Derval N, Sacher F, et al. Sudden cardiac arrest associated with early repolarization. *N Engl J Med.* 2008;358(19):2016-2023.

Case 11

PRESENTATION

A 55-year-old male with end-stage renal disease on hemodialysis and coronary artery disease (CAD) with previous coronary bypass surgery presents with sudden onset of retrosternal chest pain. It is not relieved by nitroglycerin and is persistent, with pain radiating to the jaw and left arm.

▶▶ **Presenting Electrocardiogram: Would You Activate the Cath Lab?**

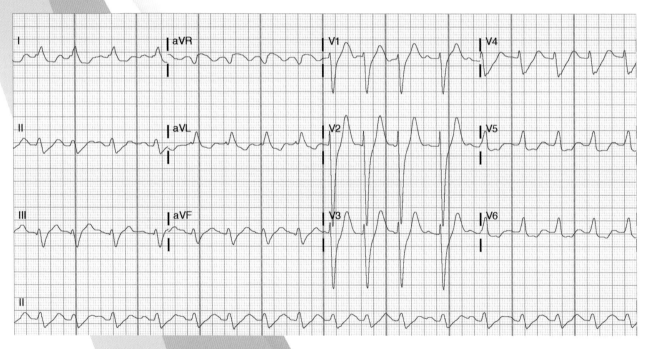

ECG 11.1

A prior electrocardiogram (ECG) is available for comparison (see ECG 11.2).

▶▶ Prior Electrocardiogram for Comparison

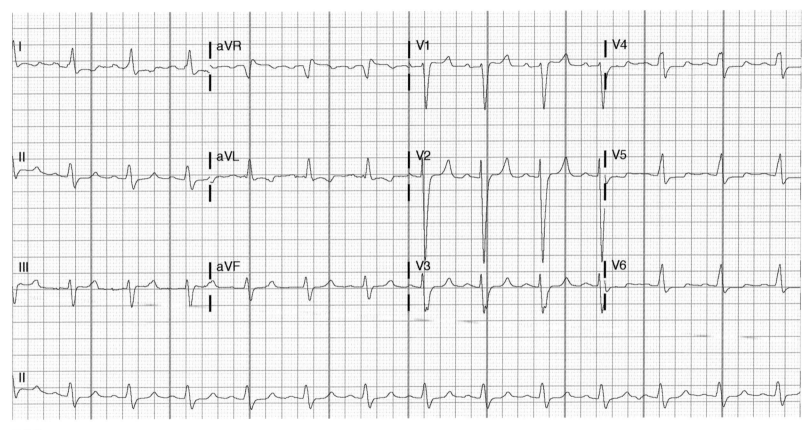

ECG 11.2

EXPLANATION

STEMI The initial ECG demonstrates sinus rhythm with left bundle branch block (LBBB). There is concordance of the anterior ST segment, which meets Sgarbossa criteria for acute myocardial ischemia in setting of an LBBB.

The patient had a thrombotic lesion of the saphenous venous graft—obtuse marginal graft (SVG-OM), which supplied a significant lateral wall territory. The lesion was ultimately treated with angioplasty and stenting.

The presence of an old LBBB often renders the diagnosis of an acute myocardial infarction (MI) difficult due to the disrupted ventricular depolarization and associated ST-T changes of repolarization. Nevertheless, derived from the Global Utilization of Streptokinase and Tissue Plasminogen Activator for Occluded Coronary Arteries-1 (GUSTO-1) trial came the Sgarbossa criteria, which is a scoring system that can help identify MI in the presence of an LBBB.[1] Its application requires the understanding of the normal LBBB repolarization pattern. **In LBBB, the ST-J point is directed in opposite direction from the main QRS vector. When the ST-J point is in the same direction as the main QRS vector (ie, both negative or both positive), it is referred to as concordant and this suggests myocardial ischemia.** The first two (of the three) items on the Sgarbossa scoring system utilize this concept.

The Sgarbossa scoring system assigns:

- Five points for ST-segment elevation of 1 mm or more in the same direction (concordant) as the QRS complex in any lead.
- Three points for ST-segment depression of 1 mm or more in any lead from V_1 to V_3.
- Two points for ST-segment elevation of 5 mm or more that is discordant with the QRS complex.

Greater than or equal to 3 points is suggestive of ischemia, and achieves a specificity of 90%, but with a sensitivity of only 36%. Note that the third criteria may have limitations when the underlying LBBB is met with left ventricular hypertrophy (LVH) or with conditions with prominent voltages.[1] Furthermore, the sensitivity of the third criteria can be improved by applying the "modified Sgarbossa" criteria, where an ST/S ratio of ≤ -0.25 in leads with excessive relative discordance suggests ischemia (ie, an ST/S ratio of -0.3 would suggest ischemia). In the original study cohort by Smith et al[2], the sensitivity is increased from 52% using the traditional Sgarbossa criteria to 91% using the modified criteria, while maintaining 90% specificity.

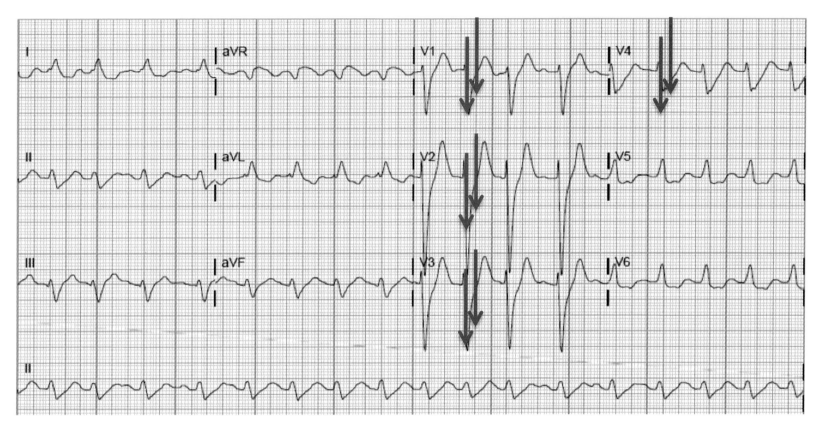

ECG 11.3

Review of the presenting ECG. Note the concordance (*red arrows both pointing downward*) of the main QRS complex vector and the ST-J point direction in leads V_1 to V_4, which is suggestive of ischemia in setting of LBBB.

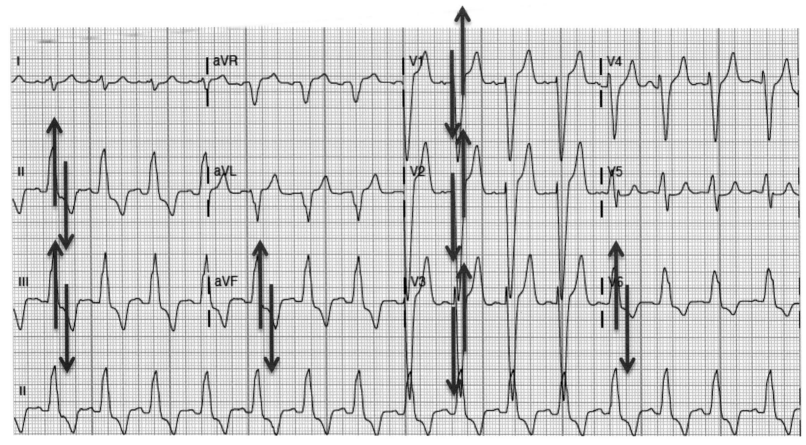

ECG 11.4

This is an ECG example of a typical LBBB without coronary ischemia. Note the direction (*red arrows point in opposite direction*) of the QRS complex vector and ST-J point direction are pointing away from each other (ie, discordant), which is a normal finding in LBBB (and of right ventricle [RV]-paced rhythm).

References

1. Sgarbossa EB, Pinski SL, Barbagelata A, et al. Electrocardiographic diagnosis of evolving acute myocardial infarction in the presence of left bundle-branch block. GUSTO-1 (Global Utilization of Streptokinase and Tissue Plasminogen Activator for Occluded Coronary Arteries) Investigators. *N Engl J Med*. 1996;334(8):481-487.
2. Smith SW, Dodd KW, Henry TD, Dvorak DM, Pearce LA. Diagnosis of ST-elevation myocardial infarction in the presence of left bundle branch block with the ST-elevation to S-wave ratio in a modified Sgarbossa rule. *Ann Emerg Med*. 2012;60(6):766-776.

Case 12

PRESENTATION

A 62-year-old female with hypertension, hyperlipidemia, and diabetes presents with chest pain. She describes constant 10 out of 10 chest pain radiating to her left arm for the past several hours. It is associated with shortness of breath and diaphoresis.

▶▶ **Presenting Electrocardiogram: Would You Activate the Cath Lab?**

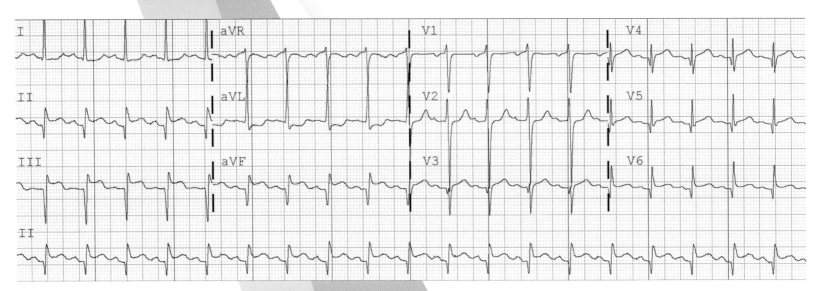

ECG 12.1

There is no prior electrocardiogram (ECG) available for comparison.

EXPLANATION

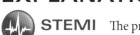 **STEMI**   The presenting ECG demonstrates ≥1-mm ST elevation in leads II, III, and aVF with consistent acute inferior ST-segment elevation myocardial infarction (STEMI).

The culprit lesion was a thrombotic 95% stenosis in the ostial right posterior descending artery, a branch of the right coronary artery (RCA). There were luminal irregularities of atherosclerosis in the remaining vessels.

Case 13

PRESENTATION

A 74-year-old male with prior coronary artery bypass grafting (CABG) more than 20 years ago and multiple coronary stents, who is undergoing chemotherapy and radiation for advanced stage 4 glioblastoma multiforme presents to the emergency department with chest pain. The patient had a witnessed seizure en route to the hospital and is hypoxic on room air.

▶▶ **Presenting Electrocardiogram: Would You Activate the Cath Lab?**

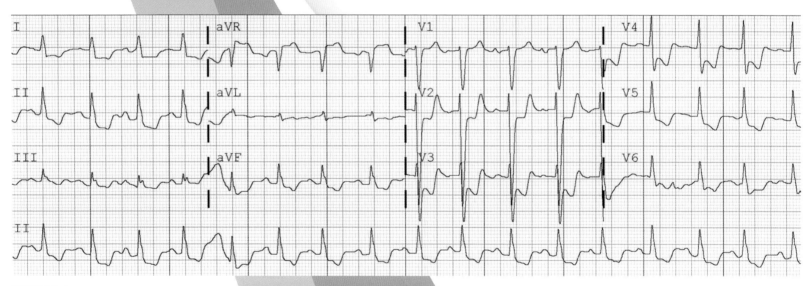

ECG 13.1

A prior electrocardiogram (ECG) is available for comparison (see ECG 13.2).

▶▶ Prior ECG for Comparison

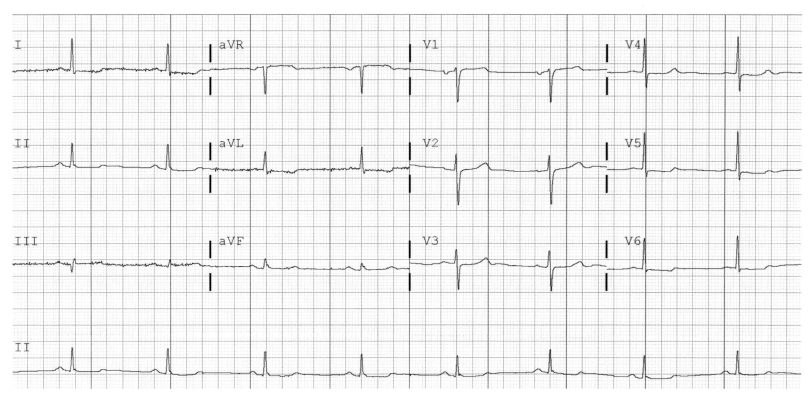

ECG 13.2

EXPLANATION

STEMI Although the ECG does not meet the criteria for ST-elevation myocardial infarction (STEMI), given the diffuse ST depressions indicating severe multivessel disease, the cardiac catheterization team was activated.

After discussion with the patient's family, no cardiac catheterization was performed. The patient had a grave overall prognosis and was truly "too sick" to undergo a cardiac catheterization. Although he may have had severe acute coronary artery disease, his active medical issues included advanced malignancy, seizure, and hypoxia.

Rushing a patient like this to the catheterization laboratory may cause more harm than good. Remember to recognize the big picture of the patient's clinical condition, even when timely clinical decisions are necessary. Awareness of the risk–benefit ratio, which may entail emergent consultation with cardiology to assist in determining, needs to be considered.

Coronary angioplasty, which would involve dual antiplatelet therapy and full dose intraprocedural anticoagulation, would subject the patient to an extremely high risk of intracranial bleeding. Brain tumors that are most likely to bleed include primary brain tumors such as glioblastoma multiforme, and metastatic brain tumors of papillary thyroid, melanoma, and renal cell carcinoma, as well as the more common cancers of lung and breast.[1]

Reference

1. Velander AJ, DeAngelis LM, Navi BB. Intracranial hemorrhage in patients with cancer. *Curr Atheroscler Rep.* 2012;14(4):373-381. doi:10.1007/s11883-012-0250-3.

Case 14

PRESENTATION

A 69-year-old male with end-stage renal disease on hemodialysis, diabetes, hyperlipidemia, and hypertension presents with an episode of "stabbing" right-sided chest pain that radiated to the back. He states it worsened when lying flat, and was associated with nausea and vomiting.

▸▸ **Presenting Electrocardiogram: Would You Activate the Cath Lab?**

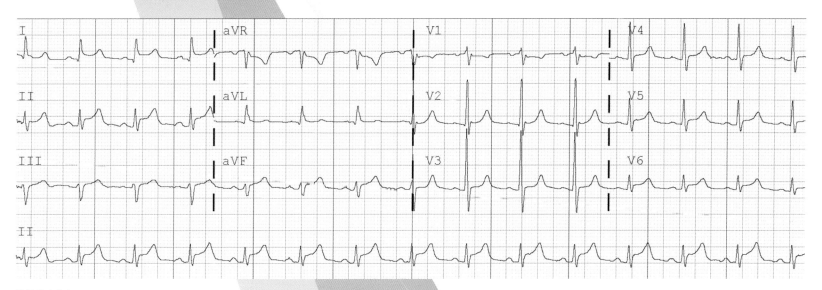

ECG 14.1

A prior electrocardiogram (ECG) is available for comparison (see ECG 14.2).

▶▶ Prior Electrocardiogram for Comparison

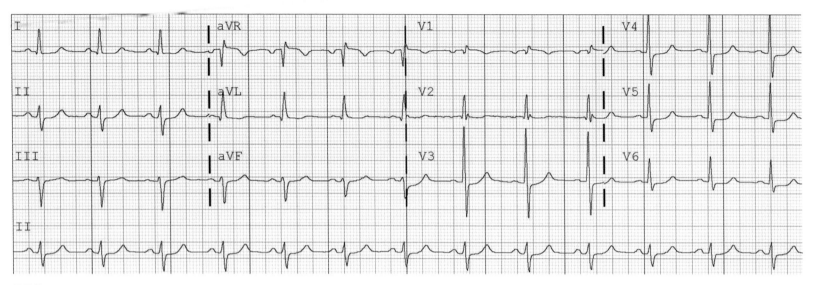

ECG 14.2

EXPLANATION

STEMI   The presenting ECG demonstrates an inferolateral ST-segment elevation myocardial infarction (STEMI), with ≥1 mm in leads II, III, aVF (inferior) as well as leads V_5 and V_6 (lateral).

Despite the relatively atypical presentation of the patient's chest pain symptoms, there was a culprit 100% proximal left circumflex coronary artery (LCx) lesion.

A popular question that often arises with inferior wall myocardial infarctions (MI) is how to determine whether the right coronary artery (RCA) or the LCx is the culprit. A useful way but not perfect method is to compare the height of the ST elevations in leads II and III. LCx occlusions tend to have elevated ST segments in lead II > lead III, as in this case. Accuracy of this common teaching is limited by patient-to-patient variation in coronary anatomy (ie, vessel size and vessel course), site of the culprit lesions (ie, proximal, mid, or distal segment of the vessel), ECG lead placement, and position of the patient's heart.

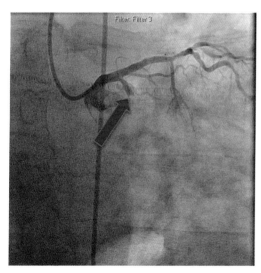 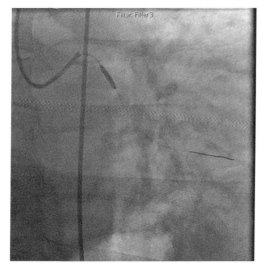 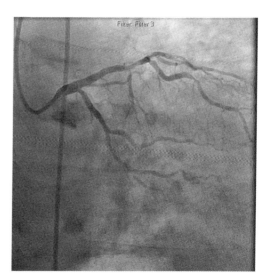

Figure 14.1   **Figure 14.2**   **Figure 14.3**

Culprit lesion with 100% stenosis in the proximal LCx (*Figure 14.1; red arrow*), treated with balloon angioplasty and stenting; Figures 14.1 to 14.3.

Case 15

PRESENTATION

A 69-year-old female with a hematologic malignancy presents for a placement of a chest wall infusion catheter for planned chemotherapy. Soon after the procedure, the patient developed severe chest pain and was brought to the emergency department for further evaluation. On arrival, she was diaphoretic and clearly in distress.

Vital signs were stable despite her unwell appearance. X-ray excluded pneumothorax and other acute lung pathology.

▸▸ **Presenting Electrocardiogram: Would You Activate the Cath Lab?**

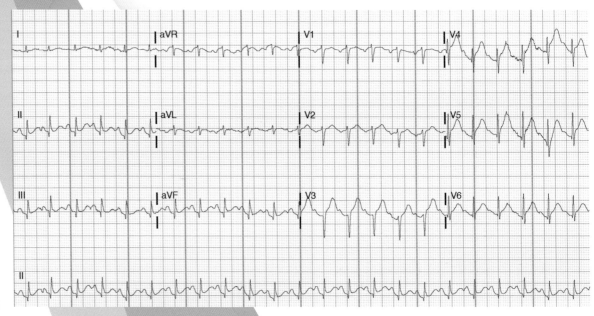

ECG 15.1

A prior electrocardiogram (ECG) is available for comparison (see ECG 15.2).

▶▶ Prior Electrocardiogram for Comparison

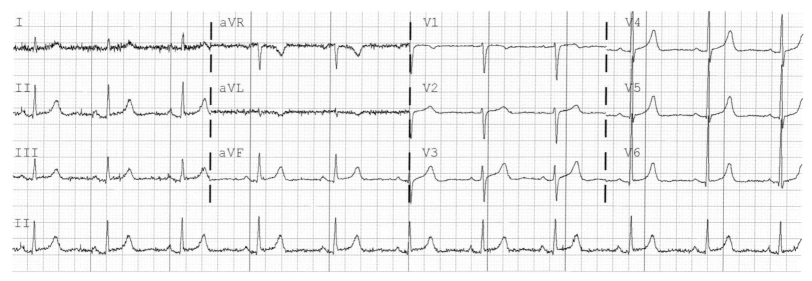

ECG 15.2

EXPLANATION

FEMI The presenting ECG demonstrates sinus tachycardia with broad hyperacute T waves with anterolateral ST elevations; however, cardiac catheterization revealed only mild atherosclerosis—without acute coronary lesions.

This was a case of stress-induced cardiomyopathy (Takotsubo cardiomyopathy). The patient's left ventricle (LV) function noted on ventriculogram was severely depressed with the classic apical ballooning pattern. Dynamic ECG changes are known to occur in cases of stress-induced cardiomyopathy, often mimicking the ST elevations of true myocardial ischemia.[1] Stress-induced cardiomyopathy remains a diagnosis of exclusion, and coronary angiogram is still necessary to confirm the diagnosis.

It is conceivable that the chest wall infusion port catheter placement was the "stressor" that triggered the acute cardiomyopathy and ECG changes. According to The International Takotsubo Registry, >70% of cases can be linked to an identifiable emotional or physical stressor. Although most cases of LV dysfunction fully recover over a matter of days to weeks, there is a substantial risk of hypotension, cardiogenic shock, pulmonary edema, and even death during the active phase of the cardiomyopathy. The morbidity may result from either the cardiomyopathy itself or from the underlying stressor (ie, sepsis, other acute illness, etc).[1]

Noteworthy is the evolving ECG pattern over the next several days to weeks, which may be seen as part of the natural history of this form of cardiomyopathy (see subsequent ECGs); these changes mimic ischemic ECG changes.

Repeat ECG *1 day* after symptom onset (ECG 15.3).

Development of the characteristic QT prolongation with deep T-wave inversions, which in isolation would be concerning for ischemia.

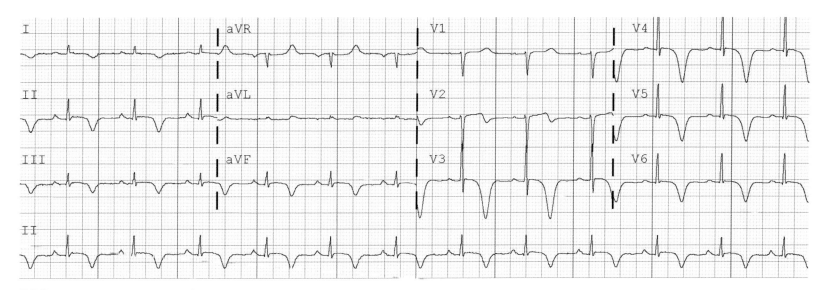

ECG 15.3

Repeat ECG *4 days* after symptom onset (ECG 15.4).

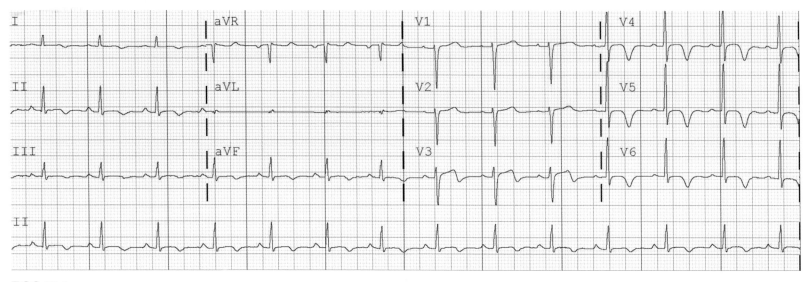

ECG 15.4

Regression of the QT prolongation and deep T-wave inversions becomes biphasic. Again, in isolation, these "ischemia" ST changes persist.

Repeat ECG *3 weeks* after symptom onset (ECG 15.5).

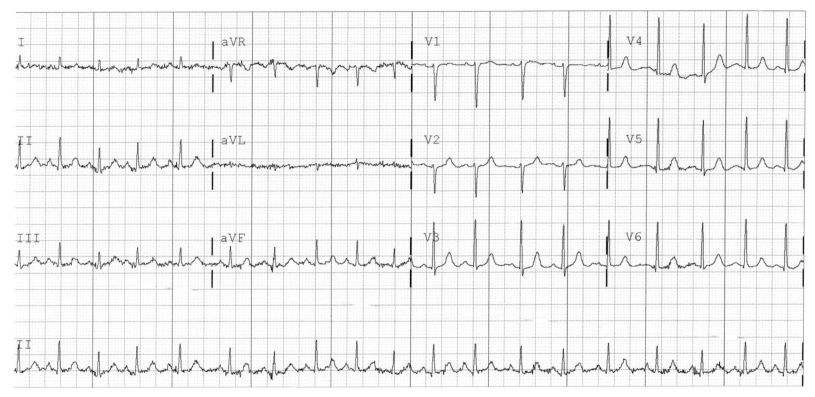

ECG 15.5

Return to baseline ST-T pattern. Repeat echocardiogram also revealed normal ventricular function.

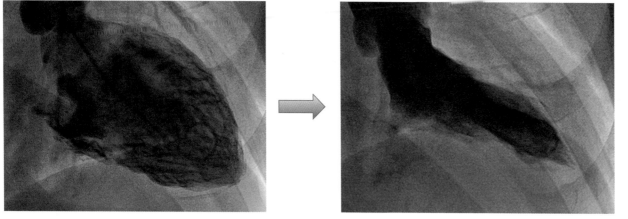

Figure 15.1

Figure 15.2

Illustrated is the left ventricle during diastole (*Figure 15.1*) and during systole (*Figure 15.2*). Notice the symmetrical inward contraction of the normal functioning left ventricle (*Figure 15.3*).

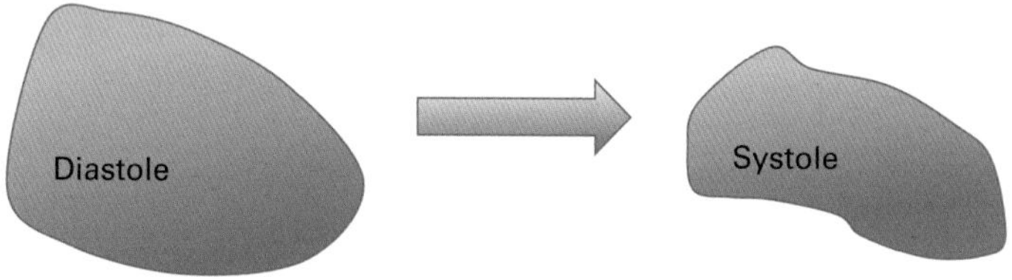

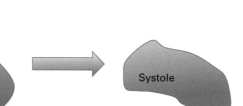

Diastole

Systole

Figure 15.3

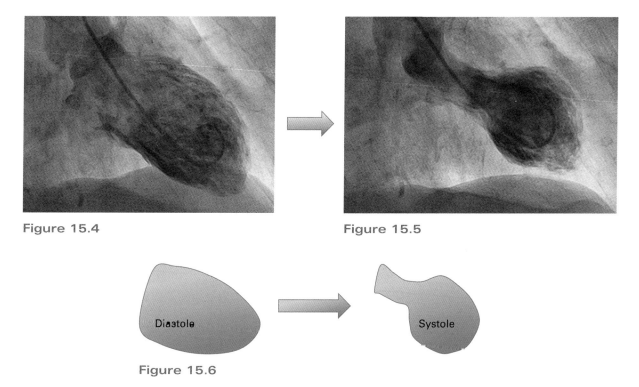

Figure 15.4

Figure 15.5

Figures 15.4 to 15.6. Illustrated is a ventriculogram demonstrating Takotsubo's cardiomyopathy, or apical ballooning syndrome demonstrated by the patient in Case 15. The distal portion of the ventricle does not contract and actually "balloons" outward during systole.

Figure 15.6

Reference

1. Templin C, Ghadri JR, Diekmann J, et al. Clinical features and outcomes of Takotsubo (stress) cardiomyopathy. *N Engl J Med.* 2015;373(10):929-938.

Case 16

PRESENTATION

A 42-year-old male with insulin-dependent diabetes and hypertension presents with episodes of chest pain for the past month. The pain is described as "tingling" in quality and is prolonged in duration and increasing in the recent past few days. It radiates to the left shoulder and most recently became associated with nausea and dizziness.

▸▸ **Presenting Electrocardiogram: Would You Activate the Cath Lab?**

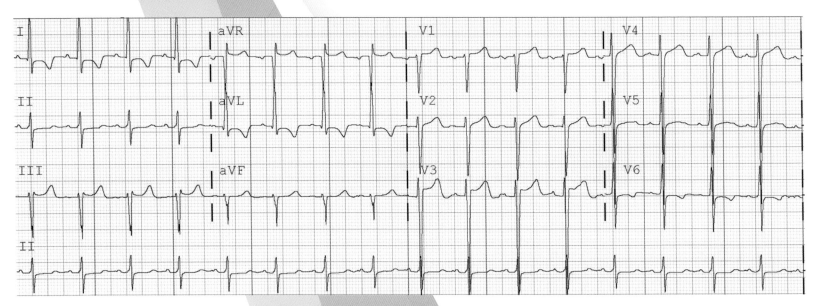

ECG 16.1

There is no prior electrocardiogram (ECG) available for comparison.

EXPLANATION

FEMI The patient's presenting ECG demonstrates sinus rhythm and left ventricular hypertrophy (LVH) with secondary repolarization. The ECG meets both "voltage criteria" for LVH (ie, lead aVL with R wave >11 mm) along with "non-voltage criteria" including asymmetric T-wave inversions in leads I, aVL, and V_6 consistent with "strain" pattern. There are ST elevations (J-point elevation) in the anterior leads: lead V_1 has 1-mm ST elevation, lead V_2 has borderline 2-mm ST elevation, and lead V_3 has ≥2-mm ST elevation.

His emergent coronary angiogram showed normal coronaries. Echocardiogram confirmed severe concentric LVH, likely as a consequence of poorly controlled hypertension.

Determining the presence of an anterior ST-segment elevation myocardial infarction (STEMI) in patients with baseline ECG with LVH pattern can be difficult. With LVH, there is often the expected exaggeration of voltages in leads V_1 to V_3, including the ST segment. Note, on standard 12-lead ECG to diagnose acute myocardial infarction (MI), there needs to be ≥2-mm ST elevation in leads V_2 and V_3 to meet American Heart Association (AHA)/American College of Cardiology (ACC) criteria.[1] LVH generally does not cause ST-segment elevations in the inferior leads, and therefore the ECG diagnosis of an inferior STEMI with LVH is generally not problematic. STEMI and LVH will be reviewed.

The first step in determining STEMI versus fake ST-elevation MI (FEMI) when faced with LVH is recognizing the expected ECG patterns of LVH. Familiarizing yourself with what is meant by "normal repolarization" and "strain pattern" can help distinguish physiologic ST-segment deviations from ischemic pathology. Most experienced ECG readers will gain a feel for what an LVH pattern should look like (of course incorporating established ECG criteria for LVH).

Commonly used LVH criteria include:

Cornell criteria: R wave in aVL + S wave in V_3 >20 mm in female, and >28 mm in male.[2]
Sokolow–Lyon voltage: S wave in V_1 + R wave in V_5 or V_6 ≥ 35 mm.[3]
Limb lead voltage criteria: R wave in aVL >11 mm. [4]
The Cornell criteria, which is regarded as the most accurate with a specificity of 90%, only has a sensitivity of roughly 30%.[5]

A "strain" pattern occurs in approximately 70% of patients with ECG with LVH. The generally accepted definition of LVH strain pattern is an ST depression that slopes down into an inverted asymmetrical T wave. The inverted T wave may have a terminal portion that has a positive deflection, often referred to as "T-wave overshoot." Leads with prominent R waves, often times leads I, II, aVL, V_4 to V_6 will often demonstrate the strain pattern.[6,7] Review the subsequent examples of the normal ST changes accompanying LVH.

Occasionally, the presence of concave ST elevations ("smiley face") may imply a nonischemic etiology. Review Case 10. However, this is not a perfect rule as LVH may have convex ("unhappy face") ST contours.

Because the voltages on ECG with LVH are exaggerated, there has been research to determine if "normalizing" the ST segment to the relative degree of voltage amplification can help improve detection of ischemia. A commonly cited work is by Armstrong et al who looked into distinguishing anterior ischemia from LVH. Their conclusion is that if the amplitude of ST elevation divided by the R-S wave in leads V_1, V_2, or V_3 is ≥25%, acute ischemia is likely. This method carries a sensitivity of 77% and a specificity of 91% in their cohort, therefore, useful but by no means a perfect method either. Adjunctive findings of ≥3 leads with ST elevations and V_1 to V_3 T-wave inversions also help determine the presence of ischemia.[8]

▶▶ LVH Example 1

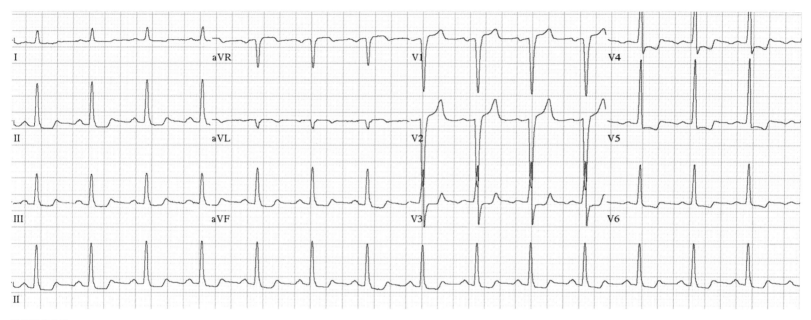

ECG 16.2

The ECG demonstrates LVH where the S wave in V_1 + R wave in V_5 is >35 mV. Note the "strain pattern," with the characteristic T-wave overshoot (ECG 16.2). In this ECG, the J-point elevation causing ST elevations in leads V_1 and V_2 may be mistaken for a STEMI.

▶▶ LVH Example 2

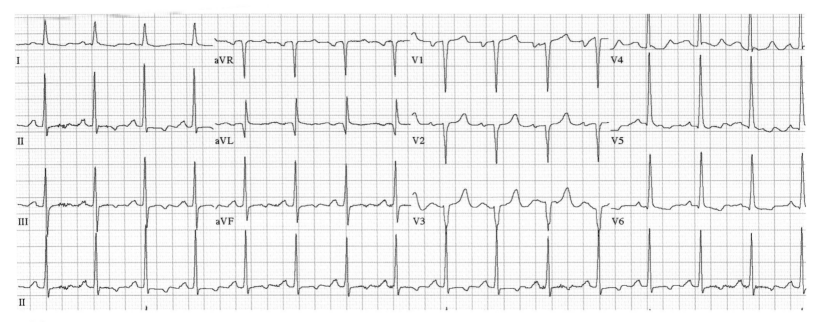

ECG 16.3

LVH pattern without ST elevation (ECG 16.3). Note the strain pattern exhibited in the inferior and lateral leads; the strain pattern is often present where the R waves are more prominent.

▶▶ LVH Example 3

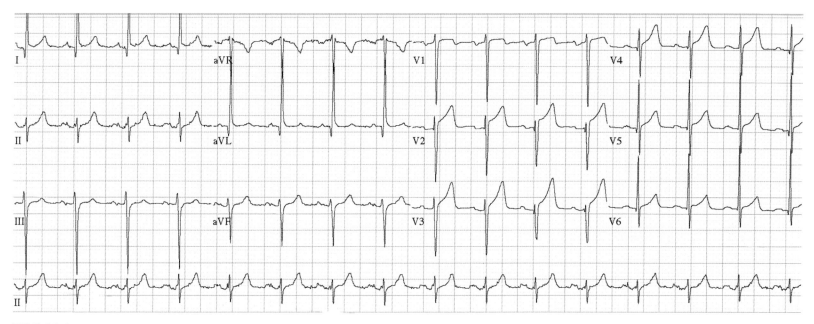

ECG 16.4

This ECG meets several LVH criteria with lead aVL ≥11 mV, the Cornell criteria of R wave in aVL + S wave in V_3 > 28 mV (in a male patient; if female, the patient would need a cutoff of >20 mV), and the Sokolow–Lyon criteria (S wave in V_1 + R wave in V_5 or V_6 ≥ 35 mm). Despite the clear >2-mm ST elevations in leads V_2 and V_3, this ECG is not indicative of ischemia. This is because the V_2 and V_3 ST elevations are not "significant enough" in relationship to the global exaggeration of voltages with LVH. From an objective standpoint, the ST-elevation amplitude divided by the RS wave in leads V_1, V_2, and V_3 is <25%, therefore not suggestive of infarction.[8]

▶▶ LVH Example 4

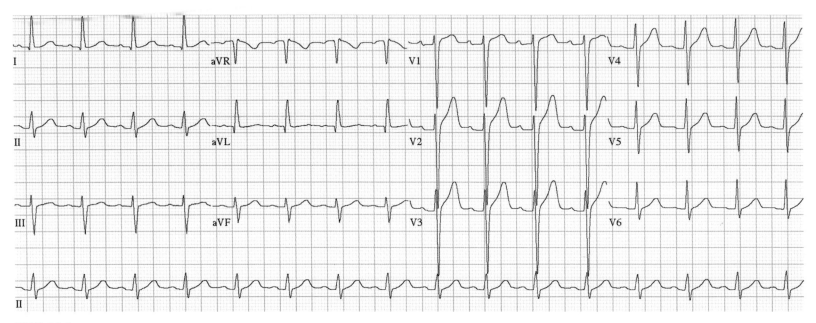

ECG 16.5

The ECG demonstrates LVH and with 2-mm ST elevations in leads V_1 to V_3 (ECG 16.5). The ST contour is concave ("smiley face") and the ST elevation amplitude divided by the RS wave in leads V_1, V_2, or V_3 is <25%, overall not suggestive of vessel occlusion.[8]

References

1. Wagner GS, Macfarlane P, Wellens H, et al.; American Heart Association Electrocardiography and Arrhythmias Committee, Council on Clinical Cardiology; American College of Cardiology Foundation; Heart Rhythm Society. AHA/ACCF/HRS recommendations for the standardization and interpretation of the electrocardiogram: part VI: acute ischemia/

infarction: a scientific statement from the American Heart Association Electrocardiography and Arrhythmias Committee, Council on Clinical Cardiology; the American College of Cardiology Foundation; and the Heart Rhythm Society. Endorsed by the International Society for Computerized Electrocardiology. *J Am Coll Cardiol.* 2009;53(11):1003-1011. doi:10.1016/j.jacc.2008.12.016.

2. Casale PN, Devereux RB, Alonso DR, Campo E, Kligfield P. Improved sex-specific criteria of left ventricular hypertrophy for clinical and computer interpretation of electrocardiograms: validation with autopsy findings. *Circulation.* 1987;75(3):565-572.

3. Sokolow M, Lyon TP. The ventricular complex in left ventricular hypertrophy as obtained by unipolar precordial and limb leads. *Am Heart J.* 1949;37(2):161-186.

4. Hancock EW, Deal BJ, Mirvis DM, et al.; American Heart Association Electrocardiography and Arrhythmias Committee, Council on Clinical Cardiology; American College of Cardiology Foundation; Heart Rhythm Society. AHA/ACCF/HRS recommendations for the standardization and interpretation of the electrocardiogram: part V: electrocardiogram changes associated with cardiac chamber hypertrophy: a scientific statement from the American Heart Association Electrocardiography and Arrhythmias Committee, Council on Clinical Cardiology; the American College of Cardiology Foundation; and the Heart Rhythm Society. Endorsed by the International Society for Computerized Electrocardiology. *J Am Coll Cardiol.* 2009;53(11):992-1002.

5. Schillaci G, Verdecchia P, Borgioni C, et al. Improved electrocardiographic diagnosis of left ventricular hypertrophy. *Am J Cardiol.* 1994;74(7):714-719.

6. Brady WJ, Chan TC, Pollack M. Electrocardiographic manifestations: patterns that confound the EKG diagnosis of acute myocardial infarction-left bundle branch block, ventricular paced rhythm, and left ventricular hypertrophy. *J Emerg Med.* 2000;18(1):71-78.

7. Sundström J, Lind L, Arnlöv J, Zethelius B, Andrén B, Lithell HO. Echocardiographic and electrocardiographic diagnoses of left ventricular hypertrophy predict mortality independently of each other in a population of elderly men. *Circulation.* 2001;103(19):2346-2351.

8. Armstrong EJ, Kulkarni AR, Bhave PD, et al. Electrocardiographic criteria for ST-elevation myocardial infarction in patients with left ventricular hypertrophy. *Am J Cardiol.* 2012;110(7):977-983.

Case 17

PRESENTATION

A 59-year-old male with former cocaine abuse presents with acute substernal chest pain, stabbing, with 8 out of 10 on the pain scale. It occurred while he was at home at rest. He still uses tobacco but does not have any known cardiac disease.

▸▸ **Presenting Electrocardiogram: Would You Activate the Cath Lab?**

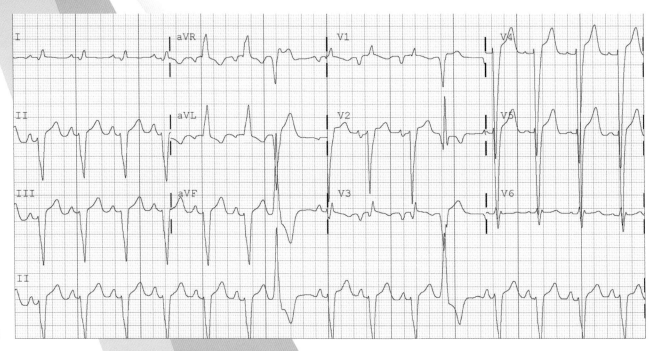

ECG 17.1

There is no prior electrocardiogram (ECG) available for comparison.

EXPLANATION

FEMI   The ECG shows sinus rhythm with frequent premature ventricular contractions (PVCs) and wide QRS complexes of approximately 140 ms consistent with nonspecific intraventricular conduction delay (IVCD). There is an ST elevation in contiguous leads in the anterior and inferior territories—which technically meets standard ST-segment elevation myocardial infarction (STEMI) criteria. However, the changes are reflective of IVCD, rather than an acute coronary syndrome.

This ECG is also notable for reversal of leads V_2 and V_3, as evidenced by the inappropriate P- and R-wave progression.

IVCD can make the diagnosis of an acute myocardial infarction (MI) difficult, especially when no previous ECG is available for comparison. In addition, the presence of IVCD can limit the accuracy of diagnosing concomitant left ventricular hypertrophy (LVH).[1]

With convincing acute chest pain symptoms, frequent ventricular ectopy (which can theoretically classify the patient as "electrically unstable"), and without obvious contraindications, a cardiac catheterization would be reasonable. In this case, the urgent catheterization did not reveal acute or high-grade coronary lesions.

IVCD, similar to left bundle branch block (LBBB), has been increasingly recognized as a marker of mortality, cardiac death, and arrhythmic death in a general population. IVCD (much like LBBB and right bundle branch block [RBBB]) is in large the end pathophysiologic process of several combined cardiac disorders including scarring, ischemia, fibrosis, and conduction degeneration.[2] On echocardiogram, the patient had severe biventricular dysfunction. He ultimately went on to receive optimal medical therapy for his newly diagnosed end-stage nonischemic cardiomyopathy.

IVCD is defined as QRS complex >110 ms that does not have morphological features consistent with either:

- LBBB (upright, monophasic QRS in left-sided leads I and V_6—and a predominantly negative QRS in right-sided lead V_1), or
- RBBB (an rSR′ complex in right-sided lead V_1—and wide terminal S waves in left-sided leads I and V_6).[3]

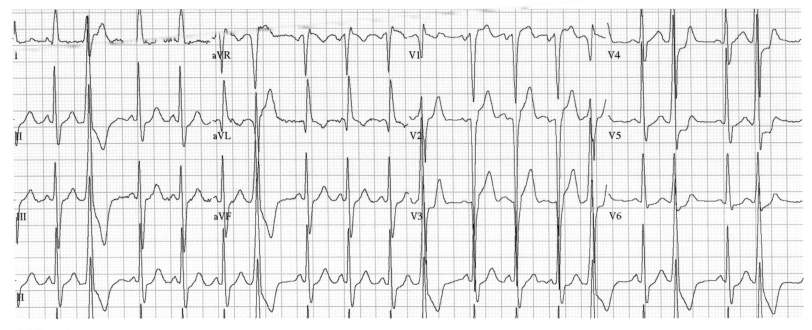

ECG 17.2

This ECG is of a patient with similar chest pain presentation as the one in this Case 17 (ECG 17.2). Likewise, this ECG has ST elevations with prominent voltages of LVH and criteria for IVCD. Both LVH and IVCD can be expected to give rise to anterior J point/ST elevations and exaggerated voltages. Cardiac catheterization was avoided in this case with recognition of the LVH/IVCD pattern.

References

1. Hancock EW, Deal BJ, Mirvis DM, et al.; American Heart Association Electrocardiography and Arrhythmias Committee, Council on Clinical Cardiology; American College of Cardiology Foundation; Heart Rhythm Society. AHA/ACCF/HRS recommendations for the standardization and interpretation of the electrocardiogram: part V: electrocardiogram changes associated with cardiac chamber hypertrophy: a scientific statement from the American Heart Association Electrocardiography and Arrhythmias Committee, Council on Clinical Cardiology; the American College of Cardiology Foundation; and the Heart Rhythm Society. Endorsed by the International Society for Computerized Electrocardiology. *J Am Coll Cardiol*. 2009;53(11):992-1002.

2. Aro AL, Anttonen O, Tikkanen JT, et al. Intraventricular conduction delay in a standard 12-lead electrocardiogram as a predictor of mortality in the general population. *Circ Arrhythm Electrophysiol*. 2011;4(5):704-710.

3. Surawicz B, Childers R, Deal BJ, et al.; American Heart Association Electrocardiography and Arrhythmias Committee, Council on Clinical Cardiology; American College of Cardiology Foundation; Heart Rhythm Society. AHA/ACCF/HRS recommendations for the standardization and interpretation of the electrocardiogram: part III: intraventricular conduction disturbances: a scientific statement from the American Heart Association Electrocardiography and Arrhythmias Committee, Council on Clinical Cardiology; the American College of Cardiology Foundation; and the Heart Rhythm Society. Endorsed by the International Society for Computerized Electrocardiology. *J Am Coll Cardiol*. 2009;53(11):976-981.

Case 18

A 77-year-old non–English speaking male with known coronary artery disease (CAD) presents with substernal chest pain and dyspnea. His symptoms have been increasingly noticeable with even slight exertion and although he has a "fear of seeking medical attention," he felt he needed urgent medical attention.

▸▸ **Presenting Electrocardiogram: Would You Activate the Cath Lab?**

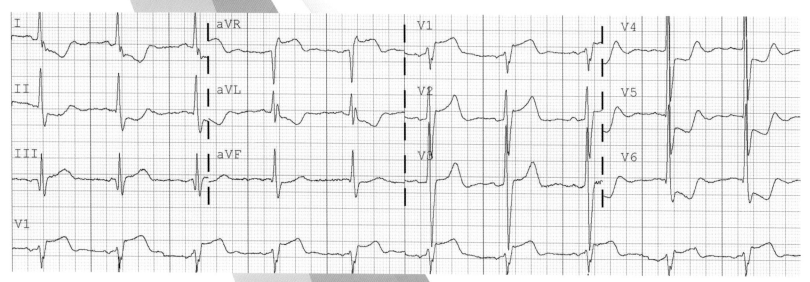

ECG 18.1

There is no prior electrocardiogram (ECG) available for comparison.

EXPLANATION

STEMI   The ECG shows >2-mm ST elevations in leads V_1 and V_2; there were also ST elevations in lead aVR, along with diffuse ST depressions—consistent with left main CAD with global myocardial ischemia. There is also left ventricular hypertrophy (LVH; ie, S wave in V_1 + R wave in V_5 is >35 mm).

The initial ECG was interpreted to be sinus rhythm and LVH with secondary repolarization and the patient was initially placed in observation. The patient did not offer any complaints (which might have been a function of his language barrier, in addition to his stoic personality). So despite the positive serum troponins, it was 24 hours before the patient was transferred to a hospital with a cardiac catheterization laboratory.

Compare an ischemic LVH to cases with LVH without ischemia; review Case 16.

As alluded to in Case 16, the presence of LVH on ECG can interfere with accurate assessment of ischemia, especially because ST elevations in leads V_1 to V_3 are expected. In this present case, even though LVH is present, there are clues that acute ischemia is present.

One critical finding is the ST elevation in aVR, which can be thought of the lead that looks "down into the chamber of the heart." ST elevation in this lead is associated with high-grade left main disease, global myocardial ischemia including severe "demand ischemia" or hypoxia. Notice the ECGs presented in Case 16, which focused on LVH, aVR is not elevated.

Another observation is that even after "adjusting for" the prominent LVH voltages, the degree of ST elevations in leads V_1 and V_2 remains significant or pathologic. In utilizing the methodology by Armstrong et al, the ST elevation amplitude divided by the RS wave in leads V_1, V_2, or V_3 is ≥25%. For example, for lead V_1, ST elevation = 3.5, and RS is 4; so 3.5/4 = 0.85, which is >0.25.[1]

The patient became profoundly hypotensive on transfer to another hospital for cardiac catheterization and died on the catheterization table because he had spiraled too far down the path of refractory cardiogenic shock to recover. The patient had an unstable 90% left main lesion, along with triple-vessel disease (stenosis in the left anterior descending coronary artery [LAD], left circumflex coronary artery [LCx], and right coronary artery [RCA]).

Patients who are not fluent in English can be the most vulnerable because of their limited communication skills. It is important to be especially vigilant when a language barrier exists.

Reference

1. Armstrong EJ, Kulkarni AR, Bhave PD, et al. Electrocardiographic criteria for ST-elevation myocardial infarction in patients with left ventricular hypertrophy. *Am J Cardiol*. 2012;110(7):977-983.

Case 19

PRESENTATION

An 83-year-old male with history of dyslipidemia, acid reflux, and anxiety presents with worsening chest pain and dyspnea for the past several hours. He describes the chest pain as pressure-like and states it worsens with exertion and radiates to his back and left arm.

▸▸ **Presenting Electrocardiogram: Would You Activate the Cath Lab?**

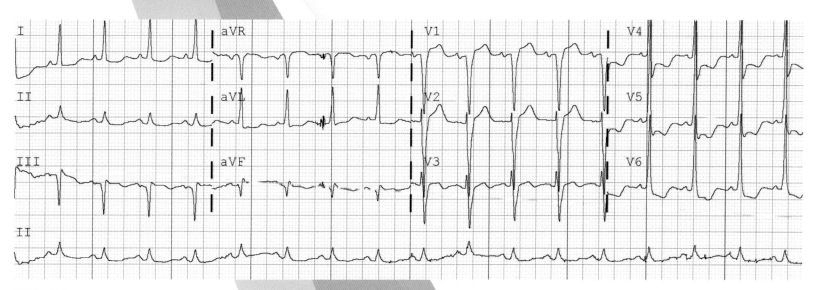

ECG 19.1

A prior electrocardiogram (ECG) is available for comparison (see ECG 19.2).

▶▶ Prior Electrocardiogram for Comparison

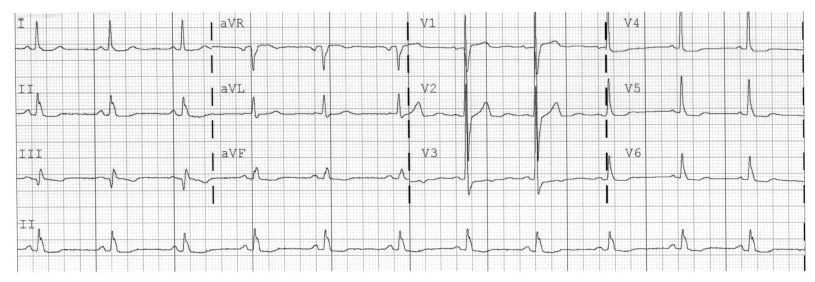

ECG 19.2

EXPLANATION

STEMI   The ECG demonstrates sinus rhythm, left ventricular hypertrophy (LVH), and $\geq$2-mm ST elevations in leads V_1 and V_2 with lateral ischemic ST changes, consistent with anterior ST-segment elevation myocardial infarction (STEMI).

The patient had a long proximal left anterior descending coronary artery (LAD) lesion with an ulcerated 95% to 99% stenosis with significantly reduced vessel flow.

Underlying LVH on an ECG makes the interpretation of an acute myocardial infarction difficult. In isolation and without a previous ECG for comparison, the anterior leads on the presenting ECG resemble the examples in Case 16, which did not demonstrate ischemia. Likewise, the lateral ST changes are very similar to a typical LVH pattern.

This case illustrates that despite using any criteria or analysis, it is often difficult to decipher STEMI versus FEMI when LVH is present. Even applying methodology from Armstrong et al,[1] which is an attempt to "normalize" the prominent voltages associated with LVH, a definitive declaration of STEMI may still not be possible, it would have been a false negative. Review Case 16.

This case shows that ECGs need to be interpreted with the clinical context. Fortunately, this patient had a prior ECG for comparison, which aided in determining the presence of an acute coronary syndrome.

Reference

1. Armstrong EJ, Kulkarni AR, Bhave PD, et al. Electrocardiographic criteria for ST-elevation myocardial infarction in patients with left ventricular hypertrophy. *Am J Cardiol.* 2012;110(7):977-983.

Case 20

PRESENTATION

A 77-year-old female with acid reflux and dyslipidemia presents with acute persistent substernal chest pain that awoke her from sleep. The pain radiated to both arms and was associated with nausea.

▶▶ **Presenting Electrocardiogram: Would You Activate the Cath Lab?**

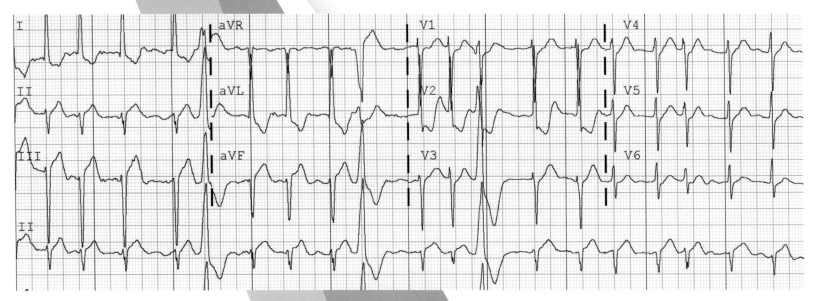

ECG 20.1

There is no prior electrocardiogram (ECG) available for comparison, a repeat ECG was performed (see ECG 20.2).

▶▶ Repeat Electrocardiogram: Would You Activate the Cath Lab?

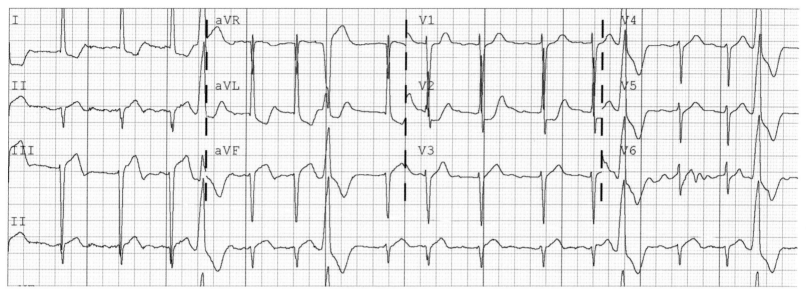

ECG 20.2

EXPLANATION

STEMI The ECG demonstrates sinus rhythm, left ventricular hypertrophy (LVH; ie, aVL > 11 mm; R wave in I + S wave in III > 25 mm), and inferior ST elevations with ST depressions in V_1 and V_2—consistent with an inferior ST-segment elevation myocardial infarction (STEMI) with posterior extension.

LVH with prominent voltages generally affects ST repolarization pattern in the anterior leads. However, inferior leads abnormalities are much likely to be pathologic, as demonstrated in this case.

Case 21

PRESENTATION

A 67-year-old female with diabetes and hypertension presents with substernal pain that radiates down to the upper abdomen. Six months ago, she had chest pain and work up included a "negative" pharmacologic nuclear stress test for coronary ischemia. At that time, she was ultimately diagnosed with acid reflux and has been on a proton-pump inhibitor. The pain is not associated with food, and occasionally with exertion and would be present for up to 20 minutes at a time.

▸▸ **Presenting Electrocardiogram: Would You Activate the Cath Lab?**

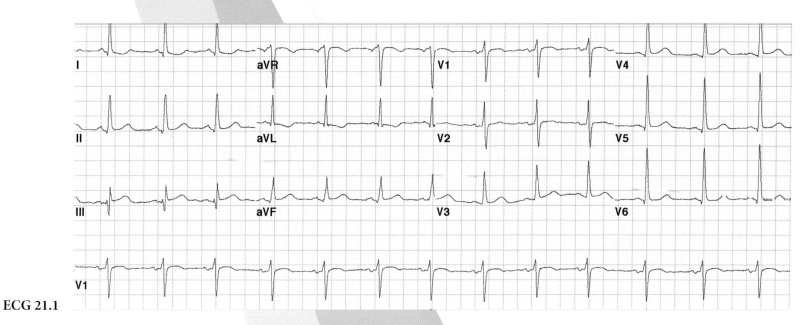

ECG 21.1

A prior electrocardiogram (ECG) is available for comparison.

▶▶ Prior Electrocardiogram for Comparison

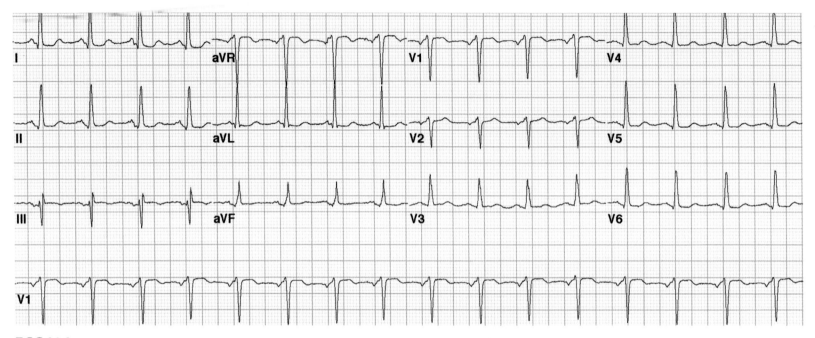

ECG 21.2

While in the emergency department, the patient reports recurrence of chest pain symptoms. Therefore, a repeat ECG was performed; see ECG 21.3.

▶▶ **Repeat Electrocardiogram: Would You Activate the Cath Lab?**

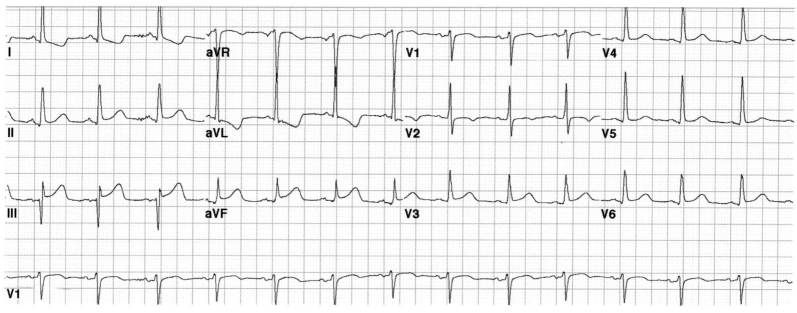

ECG 21.3

EXPLANATION

STEMI The initial ECG demonstrates 1-mm ST elevation in lead III and 0.5-mm ST elevation in lead aVF, which nearly meets criteria for ST-segment elevation myocardial infarction (STEMI) but not diagnostic. It certainly was a change from the previous comparison ECG. Note that the early transition of the R wave in lead V_2 can suggest inferior infarction. The repeat ECG was diagnostic for inferior STEMI.

In the context of the "negative" pharmacologic stress test just 6 months ago, the borderline abnormal initial ECG did not prompt activation of the cardiac catheterization laboratory. However, with ongoing symptoms, repeat ECG was performed in the emergency department, which revealed a clear-cut inferior STEMI. **Patients with ongoing symptoms should have serial ECGs to evaluate for any dynamic changes.**

Catheterization revealed multivessel coronary artery disease (CAD), with an acute culprit mid-right coronary artery (RCA) 99% lesion and was stented. The mid-left anterior descending coronary artery (LAD) had a focal 70% to 80% stenosis, and the proximal left circumflex coronary artery (LCx) had a focal 70% stenosis—both of these non-culprit lesions were subsequently stented at a later time.

A negative stress test for myocardial ischemia may have limitations in setting of severe multivessel disease (the patient had severe disease in the RCA, LAD, and LCx). "Balanced ischemia" or homogenous diseased flow can be encountered with multivessel disease and can yield a false-negative nuclear perfusion study for myocardial ischemia.[1] In essence, one would need to reconsider the diagnosis of acid reflux that she was labeled with after her "negative" stress test 6 months ago.

Stress tests are designed to evaluate the presence of obstructive lesions of roughly >70% stenosis. **Acute coronary artery lesions for most of the times occur as a result of an acute plaque rupture or plaque erosion—which are pathological processes of acute coronary syndromes that cannot be predicted by stress testing.**[2] Furthermore, the lesions that are most likely to rupture or erode are often times not flow-limiting (ie, occur in lesions <70% in stenosis severity), and therefore unable to be detected by conventional stress tests.[3] So theoretically, a patient may experience an acute coronary syndrome at any point in time, even minutes (or 6 months later as in this case) after "passing" his or her stress test.

References

1. Liu PY, Lin WY, Lin LF, et al. Chest pain with normal Thallium-201 myocardial perfusion image—is it really normal? *Acta Cardiol Sin*. 2016;32(3):328-336.
2. Virmani R, Burke AP, Farb A, Kolodgie FD. Pathology of the vulnerable plaque. *J Am Coll Cardiol*. 2006;47(8 suppl): C13-C18.
3. Stone GW, Maehara A, Lansky AJ, et al.; PROSPECT Investigators. A prospective natural-history study of coronary atherosclerosis. *N Engl J Med*. 2011;364(3):226-235.

Case 22

PRESENTATION

A 72-year-old male with coronary artery disease, diabetes, and atrial fibrillation presents with several hours of sharp, 7 out of 10 chest pain that radiates to both shoulders. There are no exacerbating or alleviating factors. The pain began during a verbal altercation with his wife.

▶▶ **Presenting Electrocardiogram: Would You Activate the Cath Lab?**

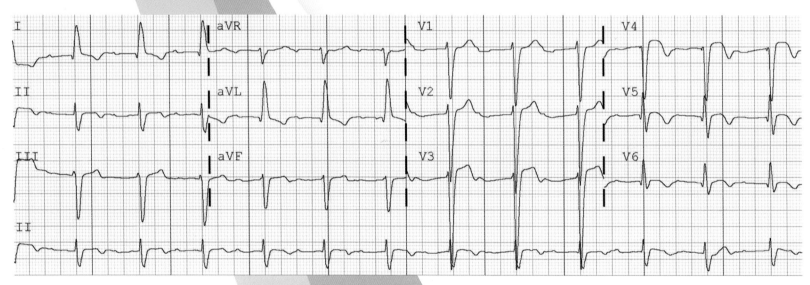

ECG 22.1

There is no prior electrocardiogram (ECG) available for comparison.

EXPLANATION

FEMI   Initial ECG demonstrates ST elevations in leads V_3 to V_5, with other evidence of an age-indeterminate anterior infarction (Q waves). However, in this case, these findings are not caused by coronary artery occlusion. Rather, the ECG findings were caused by a case of stress-induced cardiomyopathy with apical ballooning pattern, also known as Takotsubo's cardiomyopathy.

The catheterization revealed patent coronary arteries. With the patient's persistent symptoms, medical history, and abnormal ECG, a catheterization was justified. Note that emotional stress (ie, altercation with his wife, as in this case) is a typical cliché trigger for both plaque rupture of an acute coronary syndrome and for stress-induced cardiomyopathy.[1] Although there are proposed ECG criteria for distinguishing stress-induced cardiomyopathy from an acute myocardial infarction (MI), angiography remains criterion standard in the differentiation and management of these two disease conditions.[2] Review Case 15.

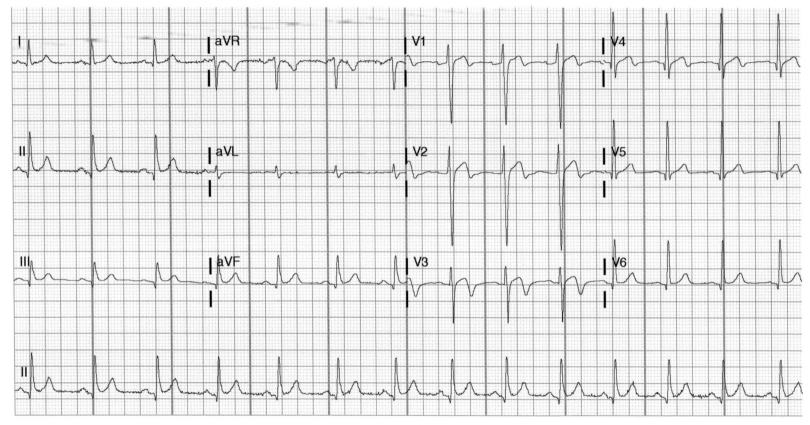

ECG 22.2

Compare ECG 22.2 with ECG 22.1. This abnormal ECG (Wellens' T-wave syndrome—biphasic/deeply inverted anterior T waves) was from a patient with chest pain due to an acute proximal left anterior descending coronary artery (LAD) lesion. Notice the similarities between this ECG (an ST-segment elevation myocardial infarction ["STEMI"]) and the example of Case 22 (a fake ST-elevation MI ["FEMI"] from stress-induced cardiomyopathy)—hence, coronary angiography is necessary to distinguish the two.

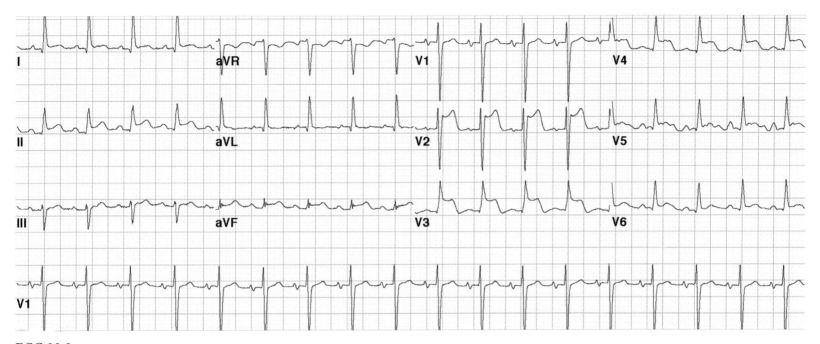

ECG 22.3

ECG 22.3 is from a patient with Takotsubo's cardiomyopathy (stress-induced cardiomyopathy) confirmed via emergent catheterization. Sometimes, it is just impossible to determine STEMI or FEMI simply by the ECG or by clinical presentation.

References

1. Krantz DS, Kop WJ, Santiago HT, Gottdiener JS. Mental stress as a trigger of myocardial ischemia and infarction. *Cardiol Clin.* 1996;14(2):271-287.
2. Tamura A, Watanabe T, Ishihara M, et al. A new electrocardiographic criterion to differentiate between Takotsubo cardiomyopathy and anterior wall ST-segment elevation acute myocardial infarction. *Am J Cardiol.* 2011;108(5):630-633.

Case 23

PRESENTATION

A 71-year-old male with a history of coronary artery disease (CAD) status postcoronary artery bypass graft (CABG) 7 years ago and active tobacco abuse presents with mid-sternal chest pain that woke him from sleep. The patient reports recent symptoms that seem consistent with unstable angina, including the need for sublingual nitroglycerin to relieve intermittent exertional substernal chest tightness.

▸▸ **Presenting Electrocardiogram: Would You Activate the Cath Lab?**

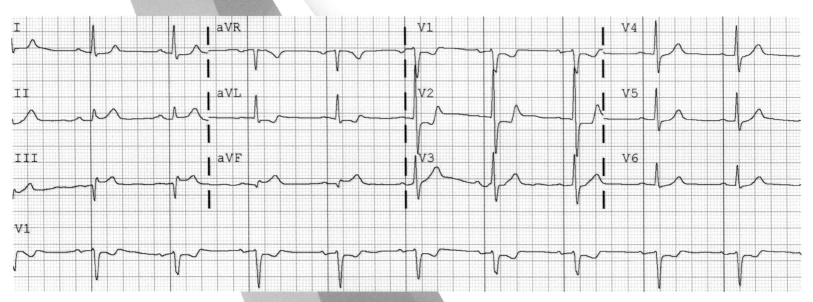

ECG 23.1

There is no prior electrocardiogram (ECG) available for comparison.

EXPLANATION

STEMI   The presenting ECG illustrates inferior ST-segment elevation myocardial infarction (STEMI; 1-mm ST elevation in leads III and aVF) with posterior extension (ST depressions in leads V_1 and V_2). Coronary angiography revealed an acute lesion in the saphenous venous graft (SVG) to right posterolateral segment that also backfills the distal right coronary artery (RCA) and right posterior descending artery (PDA) territory.

Patients with previous coronary bypass surgery grafting (CABG) may pose a more difficult emergent catheterization, especially if the native coronary and bypass graft anatomy are not known, as in this case. The culprit lesion may arise from the native coronary artery or from the surgically created bypass graft. A retrospective study of 249 patients with STEMI and previous CABG revealed the culprit vessel in the SVG in 34%, native vessel in 42%, no clear culprit in 24%, and 0% from the left internal mammary artery graft.[1]

STEMI patients with previous CABG, compared with patients without previous CABG, have a higher 5-year mortality, but this data may be confounded by more underlying comorbidities in the post-CABG patient cohort.[1] The interpretation of the ECG and acute management for STEMI in post-CABG patients is the same as for the non-CABG patients.

Reference

1. Kohl LP, Garberich RF, Yang H, et al. Outcomes of primary percutaneous coronary intervention in ST-segment elevation myocardial infarction patients with previous coronary bypass surgery. *JACC Cardiovasc Interv.* 2014;7(9):981-987.

Case 24

PRESENTATION

A 32-year-old female with hypertension, active tobacco use, and anxiety presents with persistent crushing chest pain and appears unwell. The pain is associated with nausea, vomiting, and shortness of breath. She admits to recent recreational cocaine use.

▸▸ **Presenting Electrocardiogram: Would You Activate the Cath Lab?**

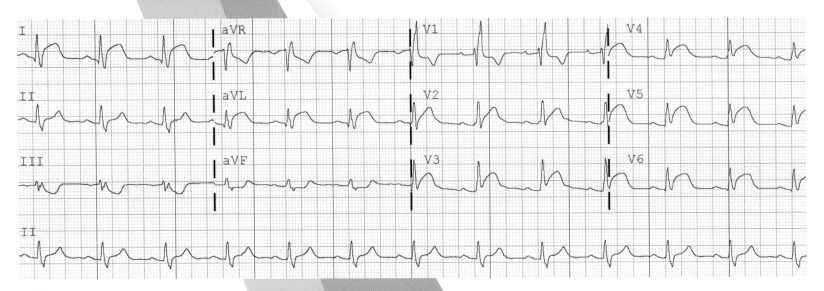

ECG 24.1

There is no prior electrocardiogram (ECG) available for comparison.

EXPLANATION

 STEMI   The ECG demonstrates anterior/lateral acute infarct (≥1-mm ST elevations in leads I, aVL, and V_3 to V_6) with underlying right bundle branch block (RBBB).

The isolated RBBB pattern typically causes ST depressions in the anteroseptal leads (V_1 to V_3). **The presence of RBBB generally does not affect the standard interpretation of ST elevations for the diagnosis of acute myocardial infarction (MI).** However, because of the disruption of the terminal phase of the QRS in the typical RBBB leads to the ST changes in lead V_1 to V_3, isolated posterior infarction (which require ST depressions on leads V_1 to V_3) may be more challenging to diagnose.

The patient had a 100% stenosis in the proximal left anterior descending coronary artery (LAD) with extensive thrombus that was subsequently treated with aspiration thrombectomy and stenting. It is often perceived that anterior MIs (as in this case) would result in a larger infarct size, and therefore have a higher chance of resulting in a left bundle branch block (LBBB). However, this is not true. In fact, RBBB tends to be associated with a larger infarct size by cardiac magnetic resonance imaging (MRI) assessment and is associated with an occlusion of the proximal LAD. LBBB tends to be nonischemic in origin, and if indeed from ischemia would require typically both proximal LAD and right coronary artery (RCA) occlusions.[1]

Cocaine-associated chest pain is due to several mechanisms. Among these include vessel spasm and hypertension due to sympathetic activation, enhanced inotropy, and heart rate, which may trigger myocardial dysfunction, and platelet aggregation leading to macro- or microvessel thrombosis and accelerated atherosclerosis.[2]

Evaluation of cocaine-related chest pain is similar to that of non–cocaine users—including ECG and standard monitoring.[3] Interestingly and important to be aware is that an abnormal ECG is commonly encountered in a significant percentage of cocaine-related chest pain cases and may lead to misinterpretation of active ischemia. For example, in a retrospective study by Gitter et al,[4] 43% in his study cohort presented with ST elevations of which only 19% were due to myocardial injury, but 58% from early repolarization and 16% from left ventricular hypertrophy (LVH). These common baseline ECG changes may reflect the younger population and the anticipated cardiac pathology associated with cocaine use.[2,4]

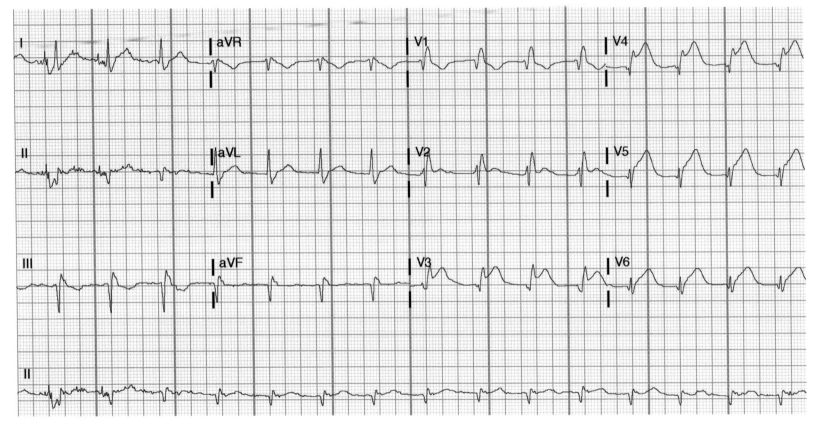

ECG 24.2

ECG 24.2 is of another patient with an *underlying RBBB*, who suffered an *anterior* ST-segment elevation myocardial infarction (*STEMI*).

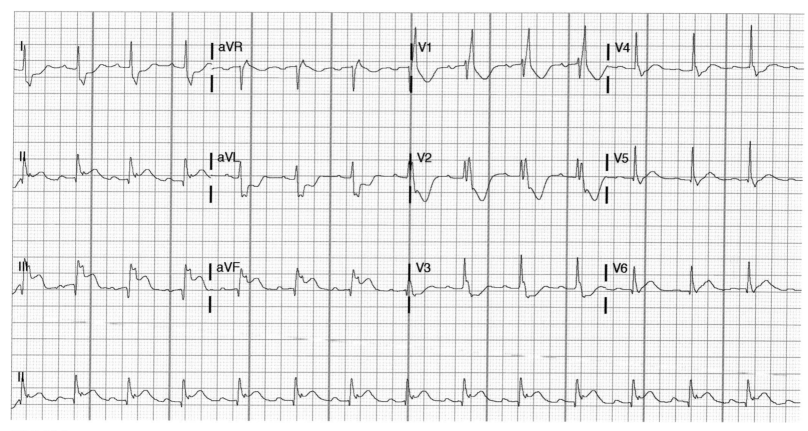

ECG 24.3

ECG 24.3 is of a patient with an *underlying RBBB*, who suffered an *inferior STEMI*.

References

1. Strauss DG, Loring Z, Selvester RH, et al. Right, but not left, bundle branch block is associated with large anteroseptal scar. *J Am Coll Cardiol.* 2013;62(11):959-967.
2. Finkel JB, Marhefka GD. Rethinking cocaine-associated chest pain and acute coronary syndromes. *Mayo Clin Proc.* 2011;86(12):1198-1207.
3. Wright RS, Anderson JL, Adams CD, et al.; American College of Cardiology Foundation/American Heart Association Task Force on Practice Guidelines. 2011 ACCF/AHA focused update incorporated into the ACC/AHA 2007 guidelines for the management of patients with unstable angina/non-ST-elevation myocardial infarction: a report of the American College of Cardiology Foundation/American Heart Association Task Force on Practice Guidelines developed in collaboration with the American Academy of Family Physicians, Society for Cardiovascular Angiography and Interventions, and the Society of Thoracic Surgeons. *J Am Coll Cardiol.* 2011;57(19):e215-e367.
4. Gitter MJ, Goldsmith SR, Dunbar DN, Sharkey SW. Cocaine and chest pain: clinical features and outcome of patients hospitalized to rule out myocardial infarction. *Ann Intern Med.* 1991;115(4):277-282.

Case 25

PRESENTATION

A 71-year-old female with history of coronary artery disease (CAD) and cardiomyopathy with an automatic implantable cardioverter defibrillator (AICD) presents with episodic left-sided chest pain. She describes the pain as being "squeezing" in quality, and states that it radiates to the neck and back. The discomfort can last for up to 1 minute.

▶▶ **Presenting Electrocardiogram: Would You Activate the Cath Lab?**

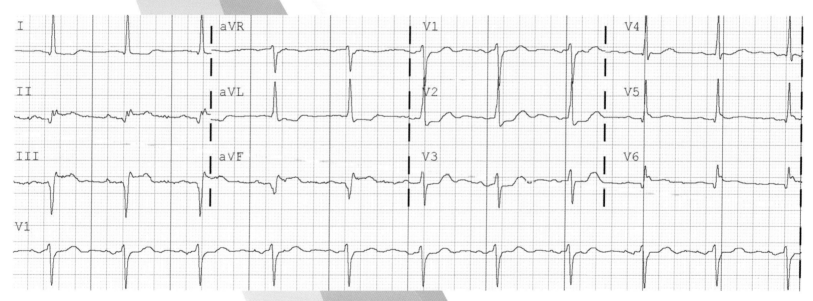

ECG 25.1

A prior electrocardiogram (ECG) is available for comparison (see ECG 25.2).

▶▶ Prior Electrocardiogram for Comparison

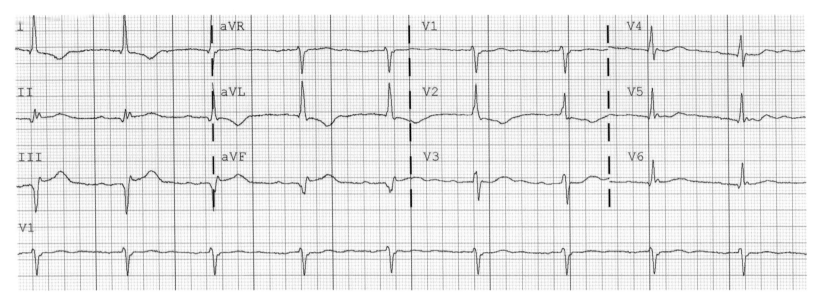

ECG 25.2

EXPLANATION

FEMI   The presenting ECG demonstrates sinus bradycardia with first-degree atrioventricular (AV) block and inferior ST elevations (≥1 mm in leads II, III, and aVF) with associated Q waves suggestive of age-indeterminate inferior infarction.

Although there were inferior ST elevations, this is the patient's baseline finding. The patient had underlying nonischemic cardiomyopathy, with notable akinesis/aneurysmal motion of the inferior and inferolateral walls. Ventricular aneurysm is a cause of persistent ST elevations on resting ECG.

A review of a previous ECG would have been handy in this case. Occasionally, it may even be helpful to provide patients a copy of their baseline abnormal ECG. The physicians did not review the prior ECGs before making the decision to activate the cardiac catheterization team. The cardiac catheterization revealed stable nonobstructive coronary artery disease.

Case 26

PRESENTATION

A 77-year-old male with lifelong active tobacco use presents with chest pain. The patient describes 8 out of 10 pain that radiates to the jaw and is associated with diaphoresis. On arrival to the emergency department, the patient is hypotensive with systolic blood pressure in the 70s to 90s.

▸▸ **Presenting Electrocardiogram: Would You Activate the Cath Lab?**

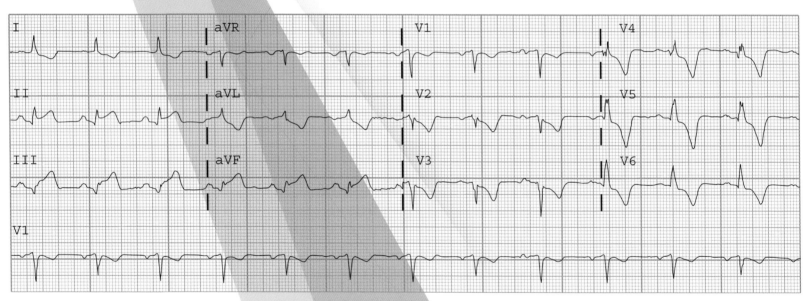

ECG 26.1

There is no prior electrocardiogram (ECG) available for comparison.

EXPLANATION

 STEMI   The initial ECG demonstrates inferior ST elevations (≥1 mm in leads II, III, and aVF) with global ST depressions suggestive of global myocardial ischemia.

This patient had an acute inferior ST-segment elevation myocardial infarction (STEMI; proximal right coronary artery [RCA] culprit), but *why such significant T-wave inversions and ST-deviations on all the other leads?*

On angiogram, the left anterior descending coronary artery (LAD) and left circumflex coronary artery (LCx) had severe non-acute occlusive disease, and the entire myocardium "depended" on the RCA. When the RCA developed an acute occlusion, the entire myocardium was in jeopardy and hence the global ST depressions. STEMIs in patients with underlying severe multivessel disease may provoke ECGs with significant ST abnormalities. This case also highlights the utility of using the ECG to risk-stratify patients with STEMIs—**not all STEMIs are created equal**. ECG clues (as in this case, with a significant ST-T change in the leads not affected by the culprit vessel) may help identify the "sicker" patients with potentially more tenuous hemodynamics. The patient required an intra-aortic balloon pump as well as intravenous pressors to achieve a better hemodynamics prior to the start of the coronary angiogram and intervention.

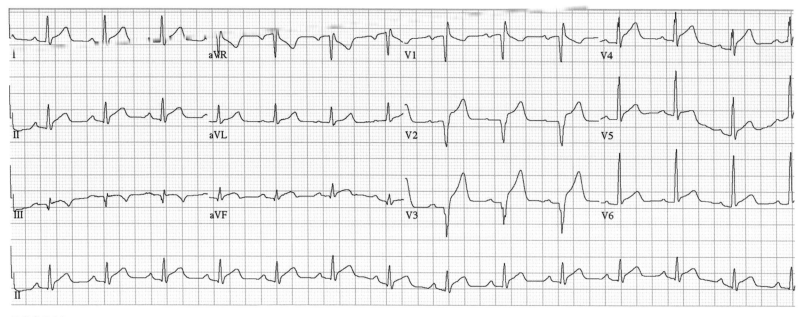

ECG 26.2

ECG 26.2 is of a patient who presented with chest pain and hypotension, with an initial ECG demonstrating ST elevations in essentially all vascular territories (inferior, anterior, and lateral). The culprit lesion was a thrombotic 80% lesion of a large RCA, which at baseline supplied collaterals to a proximal LAD chronic total occlusion. When the RCA became acute ischemic (causing inferior ST elevations), the LAD system was ischemic as well causing ST elevations in the anterior/lateral leads.

Case 27

PRESENTATION

A 78-year-old male with remote history of stenting of his right coronary artery (RCA) complains of chest pain a few hours after cervical neck laminectomy. He is diaphoretic and an electrocardiogram (ECG) was obtained.

▶▶ **Presenting Electrocardiogram: Would You Activate the Cath Lab?**

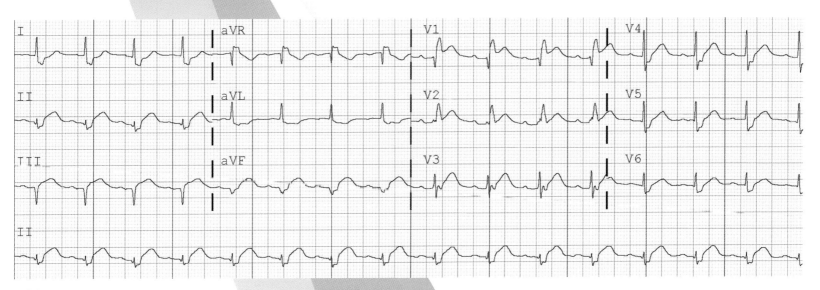

ECG 27.1

A prior ECG is available for comparison (see ECG 27.2).

▶▶ Prior Electrocardiogram for Comparison

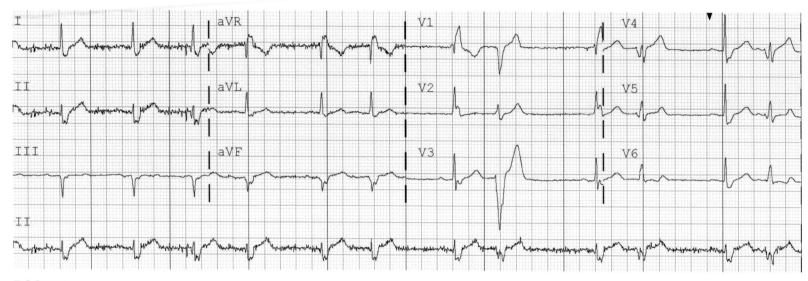

ECG 27.2

EXPLANATION

STEMI The presenting ECG demonstrates sinus rhythm, right bundle branch block (RBBB), and inferior ST elevations (≥1 mm in leads II, III, and aVF) with associated Q waves of age-indeterminate inferior infarction. There are also ST elevations of ≥2 mm in anteroseptal leads (V_1 to V_3) that are concerning for acute anterior ischemia.

This case is an example of "very" very late stent thrombosis; thrombosis of a drug-eluting stent that was placed >5 years ago, in this case to the RCA.[1] This episode of stent thrombosis was possibly instigated by a combination of the temporary cessation of dual antiplatelet therapy in preparation for his cervical laminectomy (which carries an extremely high morbidity should bleeding complications arise) and by the pro-thrombotic postoperative state.

Note, in the typical RBBB pattern, due to the delayed activation of the right ventricle, ST depressions are expected; review Case 24. Therefore, because the left anterior descending (LAD) was patent on angiogram, the ST elevation in leads V_1 to V_3 may be a reflection of the acute right ventricular (RV) infarction in setting of the inferior myocardial infarction (MI).

To an experienced ECG reader, the diagnosis of ST-segment elevation myocardial infarction **(STEMI) may be obvious, but the decision to proceed with cardiac catheterization may not always be so black and white in an immediate postoperative patient**. The bleeding risk (ie, bleeding into the spinal space by the necessary antithrombotic medications used for the coronary intervention) may outweigh the benefits of the coronary intervention. After reviewing the case with the operating surgeon, the patient underwent successful percutaneous coronary intervention (PCI) of the RCA.

Reference

1. Kaliyadan A, Siu H, Fischman DL, et al. "Very" very late stent thrombosis: acute myocardial infarction from drug-eluting stent thrombosis more than 5 years after implantation. *J Invasive Cardiol*. 2014;26(9):413-416.

Case 28

PRESENTATION

A 51-year-old male with no known cardiovascular comorbidities presents with acute 10 out of 10 crushing substernal chest pain.

▸▸ **Presenting Electrocardiogram: Would You Activate the Cath Lab?**

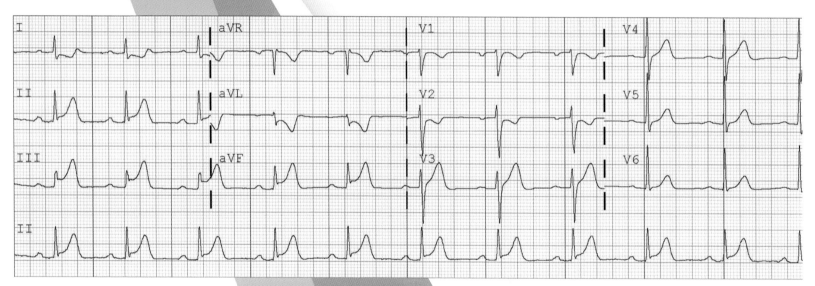

ECG 28.1

There is no prior electrocardiogram (ECG) available for comparison.

EXPLANATION

STEMI   The ECG demonstrates sinus rhythm, first-degree atrioventricular (AV) block, and acute inferior infarction (≥1-mm ST elevations in leads II, III, and aVF) with posterior extension (ST depression in lead V_2).

The patient had a 100% thrombotic mid-right coronary artery (RCA) lesion and received a stent to the mid-RCA.

There was residual coronary disease including a mid-left anterior descending coronary artery (LAD) 70% to 80% stenosis, which was deemed to be a stable non-culprit lesion and with plans for this lesion to be treated at a separate time after recovery from the acute myocardial infarction (MI).

The patient was transferred to the Cardiac Unit in stable condition. A routine post-percutaneous coronary intervention (PCI) ECG was obtained. The patient reported improved chest pain symptoms.

A routine ECG was performed several minutes post PCI (see ECG 28.2): Would you reactivate the Cath Lab?

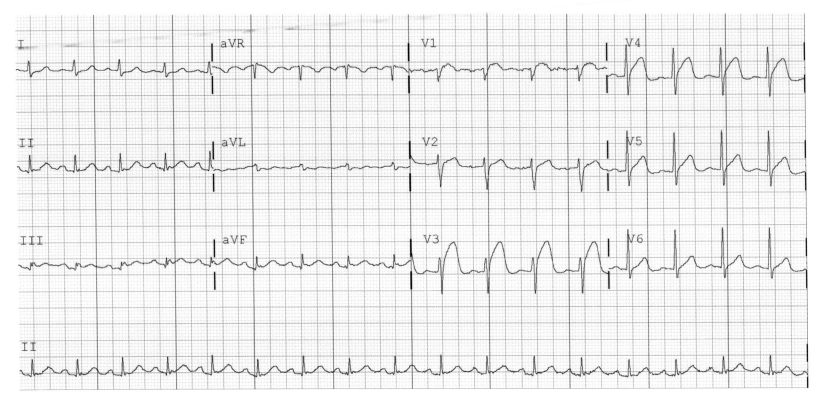

ECG 28.2

A routine post-PCI ECG was obtained: Would you *re-activate* the Cath Lab?

FEMI   The immediate post-PCI ECG demonstrated sinus tachycardia with ≥1-mm ST elevations in leads V_3 and V_4, suggestive of acute anterior injury (ECG 28.2). There is resolution of the inferior ST elevations.

However, this was a "false alert"! The patient was brought back to the cardiac catheterization laboratory, with the thought that there might have been two initial culprit lesions (ie, RCA and LAD) and that the mid-LAD needed re-inspection. However, on repeat angiogram, there were no changes to the stable appearing mid-LAD lesion and the RCA stent was patent.

In retrospect, the post-PCI ECG likely represented right ventricular (RV) infarction in setting of acute RCA disease with contribution of the stent "jail" of the second RV marginal by the end of the angioplasty and stenting. The stent in the mid-RCA had covered and "jailed" the second RV marginal (see Figures 28.1 to 28.3); the final angiogram after post-dilatation showed that this second RV marginal had occluded. Echocardiogram demonstrated RV enlargement with decreased RV function. The patient was managed conservatively at that point and the plan had remain to treat the mid-LAD lesion at a separate time.

Repeat ECG 1 day later showed resolution of the convex ST-elevation pattern in the anterior leads and subsequent echocardiogram several days later showed improved RV function. This suggests that the RV side branch may have somehow restored patency, which is a known phenomenon for side branches that were "stent jailed" and occluded at the end of the angioplasty.[1] Alternatively, the RV regained function via ample collateral circulation. Anterior ST elevations have been described in patients presenting with acute RCA ischemia, reflecting acute RV injury.[2,3]

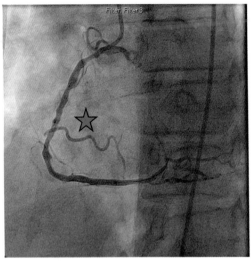

Figure 28.1

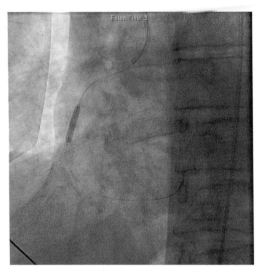

Figure 28.2

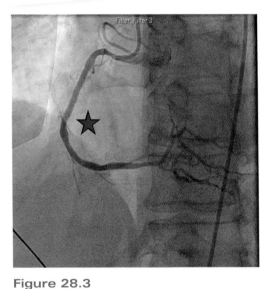

Figure 28.3

Loss of the second RV marginal (Figure 28.1; blue star) after the post-dilatation stage of angioplasty (Figure 28.2). The second RV marginal branch was occluded in the final angiogram (Figure 28.3; red star)—this occlusion likely explains the anterior ST changes post PCI, consistent with an acute RV infarction pattern.

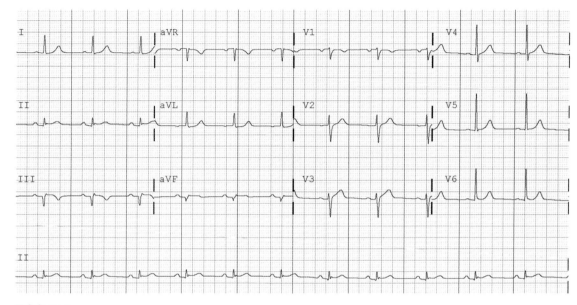

ECG 28.3

Repeat ECG performed 1 day later (ECG 28.3).

The convex anterior lead ST changes resolved without treatment of the mid-LAD lesion. This change likely reflects restored patency of the second RV marginal branch after a "stent jail occlusion or from collateral circulation revitalizing the RV function."

References

1. Fischman DL, Savage MP, Leon MB, et al. Fate of lesion-related side branches after coronary artery stenting. *J Am Coll Cardiol*. 1993;22(6):1641-1646.
2. Acikel M, Yilmaz M, Bozkurt E, Gürlertop Y, Köse N. ST segment elevation in leads V1 to V3 due to isolated right ventricular branch occlusion during primary right coronary angioplasty. *Catheter Cardiovasc Interv*. 2003;60(1):32-35.
3. Celik T, Yuksel UC, Kursaklioglu H, Iyisoy A, Kose S, Isik E. Precordial ST-segment elevation in acute occlusion of the proximal right coronary artery. *J Electrocardiol*. 2006;39(3):301-304.

Case 29

PRESENTATION

A 73-year-old female was admitted to the hospital for volume overload and congestive heart failure. The patient has dementia and is not on any medications.

The patient's blood pressure was 240/130 mmHg and was brought to the intensive care unit (ICU) for treatment of hypertensive emergency. By the evening, the patient started to "sun-down" and require intense nursing supervision due to delirium and agitation. She was suddenly noted to have tachycardia on the cardiac monitor. The patient did not report chest pain or shortness of breath. An electrocardiogram (ECG) was obtained.

▶▶ **Presenting Electrocardiogram: Would You Activate the Cath Lab?**

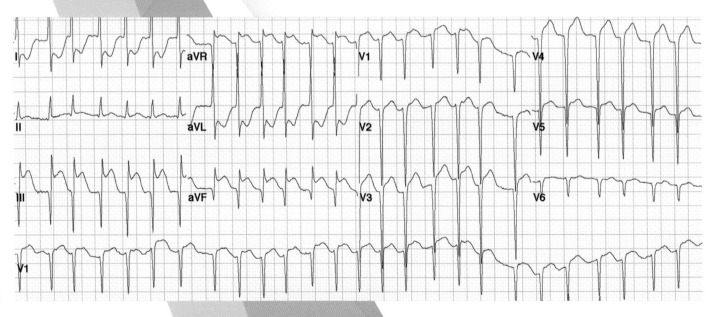

ECG 29.1

A prior ECG is available for comparison (see ECG 29.2).

▶▶ Prior Electrocardiogram for Comparison

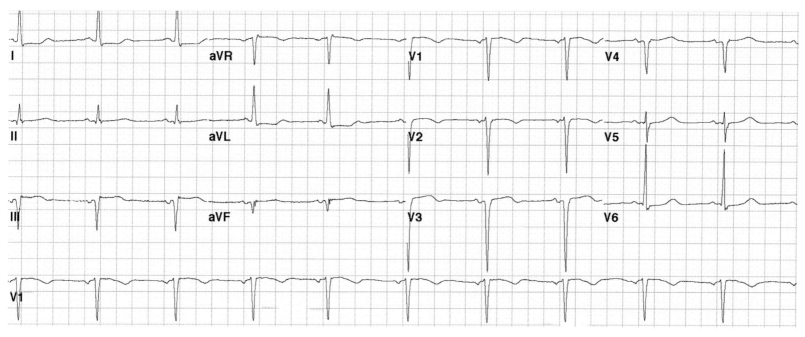

ECG 29.2

EXPLANATION

FEMI   The ECG demonstrates new atrial fibrillation with rapid ventricular response with clear inferior ST elevations. However as described later, the patient did not have an acute coronary lesion.

After recognizing the truly ischemic ECG, the next question to ask is whether the patient is a candidate for cardiac catheterization. The patient was delirious, requiring very frequent reorientation. She was unable to follow commands and would be unable to lay flat for the period of time that is required to perform a cardiac catheterization.

Intubation, in order to sedate the patient for purposes of proceeding with catheterization, is a possibility; however, this may pose more harm and there were no family members to consult with. Conscious sedation, which is the preferred form of anesthesia during cardiac catheterization, would pose difficulty in a delirious/agitated patient.

The acute delirium proceeded the new cardiac developments of atrial fibrillation and ST elevations. Amiodarone was administered and sinus rhythm was restored. Repeat ECG demonstrated resolution of the ST elevations (see ECG 29.3). When the patient's delirium was resolved, she underwent a cardiac catheterization that revealed severe multivessel disease, including a large proximal right coronary artery (RCA) with a 95% stenosis. Multivessel coronary artery disease (CAD), tachycardia from paroxysmal atrial fibrillation, and the severe concentric left ventricular hypertrophy (LVH) from chronic uncontrolled hypertension resulted in significant myocardial oxygen supply/demand mismatch and the ischemic changes on the ECG.

This case illustrates caution in performing catheterization in an uncooperative patient, which is deemed a relative contraindication.[1] Furthermore, this case shows that "demand ischemia," which usually manifests ST depressions, can also result in ST elevations in the right clinical context.

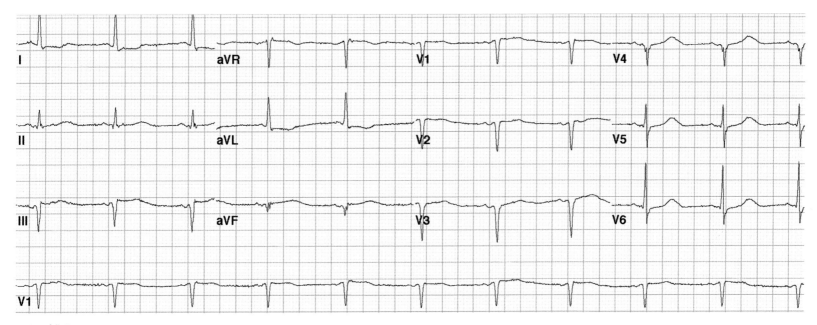

ECG 29.3

Repeat ECG after restoring sinus rhythm. Note the improvement in the ischemic changes with rate/rhythm control.

Reference

1. Scanlon PJ, Faxon DP, Audet AM, et al. ACC/AHA guidelines for coronary angiography. A report of the American College of Cardiology/American Heart Association Task Force on practice guidelines (Committee on Coronary Angiography). Developed in collaboration with the Society for Cardiac Angiography and Interventions. *J Am Coll Cardiol.* 1999;33(6):1756-1824.

Case 30

PRESENTATION

A 55-year-old female with a history of active tobacco smoking presents with acute onset chest pain that radiates to the jaw and arms.

    The triage nurse notes that her pulse was slow and irregular and she is brought immediately for evaluation.

▶▶ **Presenting Electrocardiogram: Would You Activate the Cath Lab?**

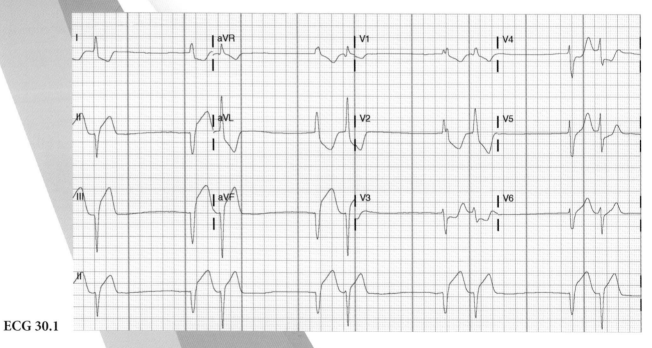

ECG 30.1

There is no prior electrocardiogram (ECG) available for comparison.

EXPLANATION

STEMI   The presenting ECG revealed sinus arrest with ST elevations seen in both the junctional escape beats and in the bigeminal junctional beats. The patient had an inferior ST-segment elevation myocardial infarction (STEMI) from a proximal right coronary artery (RCA) occlusion.

At a quick glance, the bradyarrhythmia and ectopic rhythm stand out, which may lead one to not recognize the ST elevations.

Inferior myocardial infarctions (MIs) are frequently accompanied by bradyarrhythmias including high-grade or complete heart block and sinus node dysfunction/arrest. These can arise either from ischemic injury from the infarction of the conduction system (ie, atrioventricular [AV] node and/or the sinus node) or from the heightened parasympathetic drive in setting of an inferior wall ischemic event. After revascularization, the patient's native conduction returned without the need for pacemaker support.

Case 31

PRESENTATION

A 61-year-old female with a history of diabetes and coronary artery disease with stents presents on a weekend to her local community hospital emergency department with symptoms of acute chest pain. The pain is substernal, "10 out of 10" in intensity, and is associated with nausea, vomiting, and diaphoresis.

The initial troponin was negative, and chest pains subsided after an initial round of medical therapy.

▶▶ **Presenting Electrocardiogram: Would You Activate the Cath Lab?**

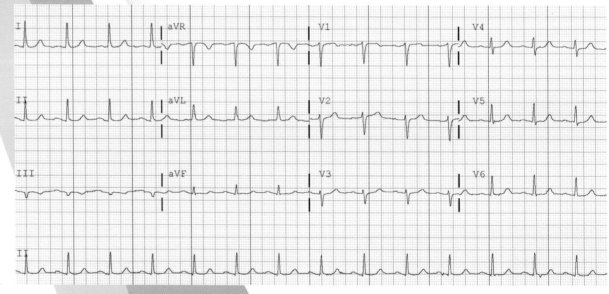

ECG 31.1

There is no prior electrocardiogram (ECG) available for comparison, a repeat ECG was performed (see ECG 31.2).

▶▶ Repeat Electrocardiogram: Would You Activate the Cath Lab?

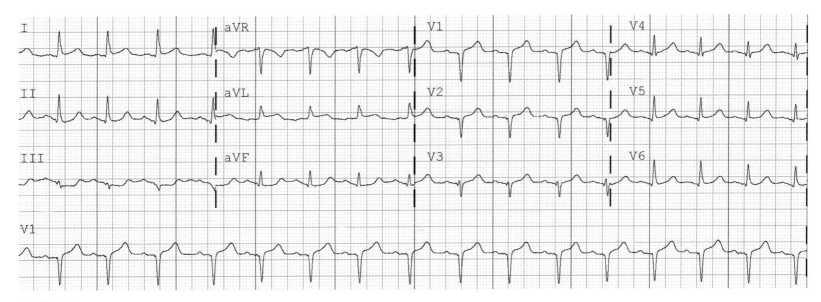

ECG 31.2

A repeat ECG was later performed, see ECG 31.3.

▶▶ Repeat Electrocardiogram: Would You Activate the Cath Lab?

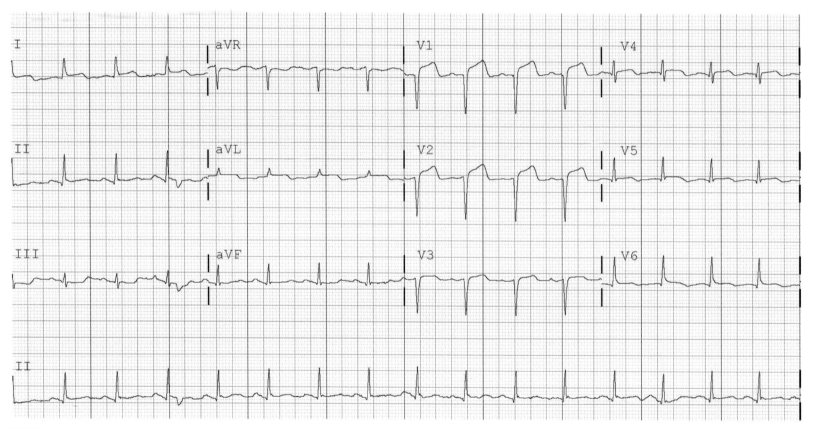

ECG 31.3

Repeat ECG was performed by the 10th hour of the patient's hospital stay.

EXPLANATION

STEMI   The initial ECG was truly normal. On the repeat ECG, however, there were new submillimeter anterior/lateral ST elevations (<1 mm in leads I, aVL, V_1 to V_6) that had developed. By the 10th hour of the hospital stay, a routine per protocol ECG was performed, and the ECG changes had become quite prominent. At that point, a second troponin T returned as markedly elevated at 27.08 ng/mL (normal range is <0.01 ng/mL).

This led to immediate attention and activation of the cardiac catheterization team.

On catheterization, the patient had an unstable lesion at the site of a previous proximal left anterior descending coronary artery (LAD) bare metal stent, and was treated with a drug-eluting stent.

This case underscores the importance of the serial reevaluation in a patient that is being managed or "ruled out" for an acute coronary syndrome; this entails revisiting the patient's symptoms, repeating ECGs, and serum cardiac biomarkers. Furthermore, some patients, as the one in this case, are not forthcoming with their symptoms and therefore close monitoring is required. The patho-physiology of an acute coronary occlusion can vary from patient to patient. In particular to this case, the gradual ECG changes noted suggest a rapidly accruing stenosis/thrombosis and potentially a moment of spontaneous vessel recanalization allowing for adequate coronary perfusion because the initial ECG was normal despite the presenting symptoms.

Case 32

PRESENTATION

An 18-year-old healthy male was admitted to the hospital with pneumonia. At 3 AM, he awoke from sleep as he developed sudden onset, unrelenting chest pain. He alerts the nurses, who found him diaphoretic and with unwell appearance.

▶▶ **Presenting Electrocardiogram: Would You Activate the Cath Lab?**

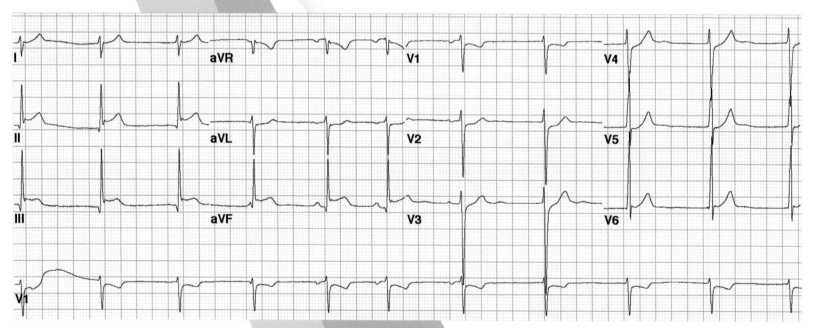

ECG 32.1

A prior electrocardiogram (ECG) is available for comparison (see ECG 32.2).

▶▶ Prior Electrocardiogram for Comparison

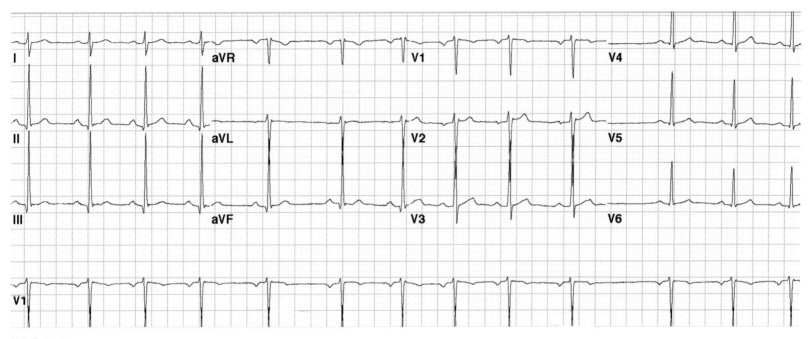

ECG 32.2

EXPLANATION

FEMI The initial ECG demonstrates sinus rhythm with ≥ 1-mm ST elevation in leads II, III, and aVF, which could be consistent with inferior ST-segment elevation myocardial infarction (STEMI) with posterior extension (ST depression in leads V_1 and V_2.

The age of the patient raised several issues pertaining to both diagnosis and management:

1. The likelihood of acute coronary disease or coronary anomaly is low, especially as the patient denied family history of early coronary artery disease (CAD) or familial dyslipidemia.
2. There are inherent risks to cardiac catheterization. An echocardiogram might be sufficient to diagnose myopericarditis and exclude acute CAD and expose the patient to less iatrogenic harm. There are, however, also logistical difficulties in arranging echocardiograms at this hour of the night.
3. There are concerns regarding the long-term effects of radiation exposure in such a young patient. Although the radiation dose can be minimized by an experienced interventional cardiologist, informed consent (perhaps involving the parents) should include disclosure of this issue as well.

After discussion with the patient and his family, a catheterization was performed. Fortunately, the coronary arteries and left ventricular (LV) function were normal. The diagnosis was made of myopericarditis in setting of pneumonia.

His troponins were mildly elevated at 0.5 ng/mL (normal range is <0.01 ng/mL), which can be expected in pericarditis and myopericarditis. Echocardiogram did not reveal wall motion abnormalities or pericardial effusion. Repeat urine toxicology was negative.

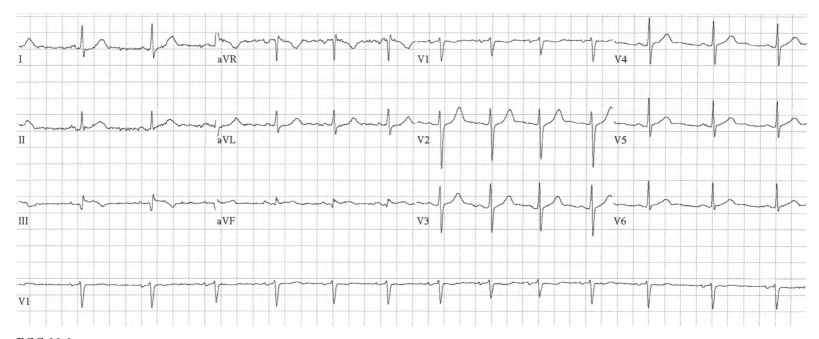

ECG 32.3

ECG 32.3 is of a young 32-year-old male who presented to the hospital with chest tightness with exertion. He had a low-grade leukocytosis and despite an abnormal ECG, and troponin I of 1.43 ng/mL (normally <0.04 ng/mL) was initially treated for pericarditis. Because of a significant family history for premature CAD, a cardiac catheterization was performed. It revealed an acute 100% mid-right coronary artery (RCA) stenosis, and high-grade non-culprit mid-left anterior descending coronary artery (LAD) stenosis as well. This case is a reminder that pericarditis is largely a diagnosis of exclusion and that CAD can affect patients at a surprisingly young age.

Case 33

PRESENTATION

A 72-year-old female with a history of coronary artery disease (CAD) with stents, as well as gastroesophageal reflux disease (GERD) presents with intermittent chest pressure for the past 3 days. She describes the pain as burning and it radiates to the back.

▶▶ **Presenting Electrocardiogram: Would You Activate the Cath Lab?**

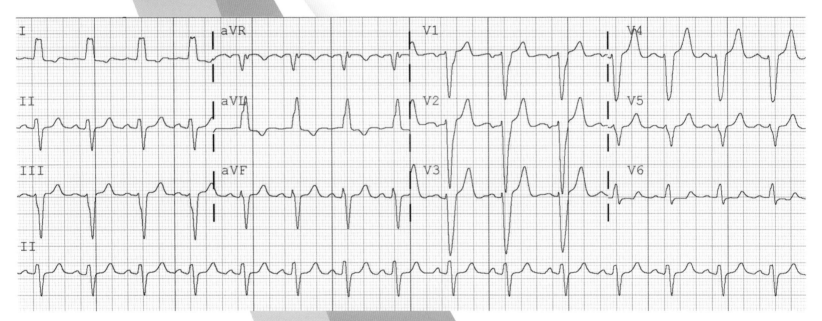

ECG 33.1

A prior electrocardiogram (ECG) is available for comparison (see ECG 33.2).

▶▶ **Prior Electrocardiogram for Comparison**

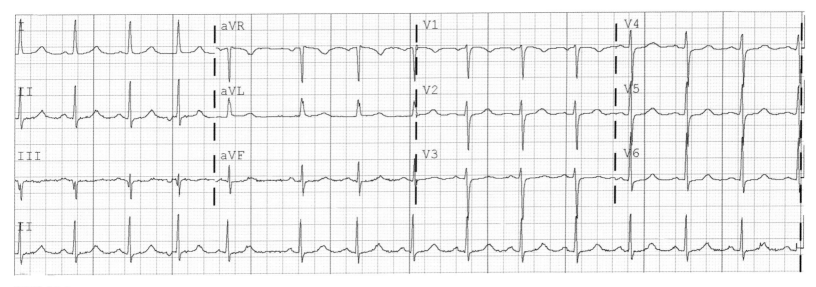

ECG 33.2

EXPLANATION

FEMI   The patient presents with chest pain symptoms and ECG had demonstrated a new or presumably new left bundle branch block (LBBB). Confusion often arises on what to do.

In the outdated 2004 American College of Cardiology/American Heart Association (ACC/AHA) guidelines for the management of acute coronary syndrome (ACS) gave a Class 1 Level of Evidence A recommendation to perform cardiac angiography in patients who presented with symptoms of ACS and a new or presumably new LBBB. However, by the updated 2013 guidelines, this recommendation has been removed.[1]

The 2004 guidelines based their recommendation on data randomized trials in the fibrinolytic era. However, review of the evidence reveals that there was a limited number of patients with actual LBBB, and furthermore, the diagnosis of vessel occlusion was based on biomarkers rather than on angiography. Clinical experience seemed to indicate that using a new LBBB as criteria for ST-segment elevation myocardial infarction (STEMI) cardiac catheterization laboratory activation led to many "false activations" (ie, no acute CAD found on emergent cardiac catheterization).[2] **Therefore, more recent updates no longer support routinely managing newly discovered LBBB as a STEMI equivalent.**

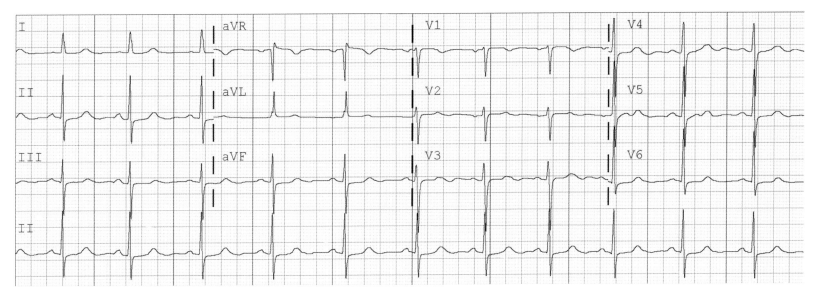

ECG 33.3

ECG 33.3 shows a repeat ECG performed the next day. Note that LBBB can be transient, as the repeat ECG no longer demonstrates LBBB. This case is an example of "rate-related" or "rate-dependent" LBBB; notice that the heart rate on the presenting ECG was faster.

References

1. O'Gara PT, Kushner FG, Ascheim DD, et al.; CF/AHA Task Force. 2013 ACCF/AHA guideline for the management of ST-elevation myocardial infarction: executive summary: a report of the American College of Cardiology Foundation/ American Heart Association Task Force on Practice Guidelines. *Circulation.* 2013;127(4):529-555.
2. Neeland IJ, Kontos MC, de Lemos JA. Evolving considerations in the management of patients with left bundle branch block and suspected myocardial infarction. *J Am Coll Cardiol.* 2012;60(2):96-105.

Case 34

PRESENTATION

A 75-year-old male with end-stage renal disease on dialysis, hypertension, diabetes, and prior stroke presents from his dialysis center with vague complaints of abdominal pain and generalized fatigue. He has chronic shortness of breath. Serum potassium and other basic laboratory testing were within normal range.

▶▶ **Presenting Electrocardiogram: Would You Activate the Cath Lab?**

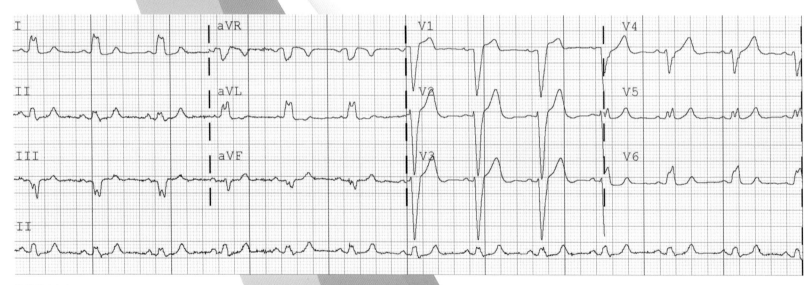

ECG 34.1

A prior electrocardiogram (ECG) is available for comparison (see ECG 34.2).

▶▶ Prior Electrocardiogram for Comparison

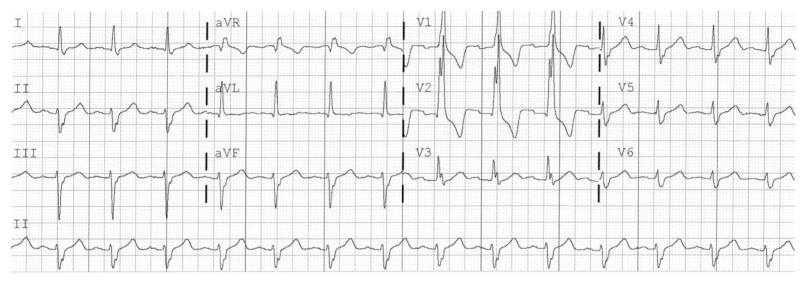

ECG 34.2

EXPLANATION

FEMI   These two ECGs illustrate alternating bundle branch block or "bilateral bundle branch block." At baseline, the patient had a right bundle branch block (RBBB) with left anterior fascicular block (LAFB), and at presentation, the patient had a left bundle branch block (LBBB). One may be quick to consider myocardial ischemia with new Q waves and ST elevations in the anterior leads, but on closer inspection, the presenting ECG demonstrates the typical pattern of LBBB.

First, as of the 2013 ST-segment elevation myocardial infarction (STEMI) guidelines, a "new or presumably new LBBB" is not an immediate indication for cardiac catheterization.[1] Review Case 33.

Second, patient's noncardiac symptoms were attributed to gastritis. However, there remains a concern that the patient's alternating bundle branch block may progress to complete heart block. Therefore, in the **2008 ACC/AHA/HRS Guidelines for Device-Based Therapy of Cardiac Rhythm Abnormalities, permanent pacemaker implantation is a Class I indication, Level of Evidence C for the management of alternating bundle branch block.**[2] The patient received a permanent pacemaker, and not a coronary angiography, after a reassuring stress test and echocardiogram.

References

1. O'Gara PT, Kushner FG, Ascheim DD, et al., 2013 ACCF/AHA guideline for the management of ST-elevation myocardial infarction: executive summary: a report of the American College of Cardiology Foundation/American Heart Association Task Force on Practice Guidelines. *J Am Coll Cardiol.* 2013;61(4):e78-e140.
2. Epstein AE, DiMarco JP, Ellenbogen KA, et al.; American College of Cardiology/American Heart Association Task Force on Practice Guidelines (Writing Committee to Revise the ACC/AHA/NASPE 2002 Guideline Update for Implantation of Cardiac Pacemakers and Antiarrhythmia Devices); American Association for Thoracic Surgery; Society of Thoracic Surgeons. ACC/AHA/HRS 2008 Guidelines for Device-Based Therapy of Cardiac Rhythm Abnormalities: a report of the American College of Cardiology/American Heart Association Task Force on Practice Guidelines (Writing Committee to revise the ACC/AHA/NASPE 2002 guideline update for implantation of cardiac pacemakers and antiarrhythmia devices) developed in collaboration with the American Association for Thoracic Surgery and Society of Thoracic Surgeons. *J Am Coll Cardiol.* 2008;51(21):e1-e62.

Case 35

PRESENTATION

A 71-year-old male with hypertension and previous cerebral aneurysm with clipping presents with intermittent chest pain over the past 5 days. The first electrocardiogram (ECG) was mildly abnormal with diffuse ST-T changes and the patient had a small elevation in serum troponin. He was subsequently admitted for observation and medical therapy was initiated for acute coronary syndrome.

While in the hospital, he had another episode of chest pain, and a repeat ECG was obtained.

▶▶ **Presenting Electrocardiogram: Would You Activate the Cath Lab?**

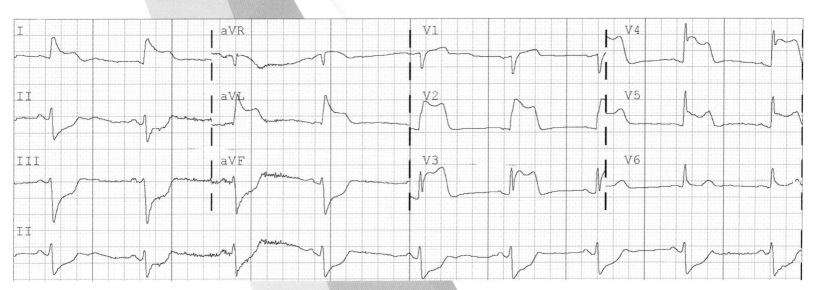

ECG 35.1

A prior ECG is available for comparison (see ECG 35.2).

▶▶ Prior Electrocardiogram for Comparison

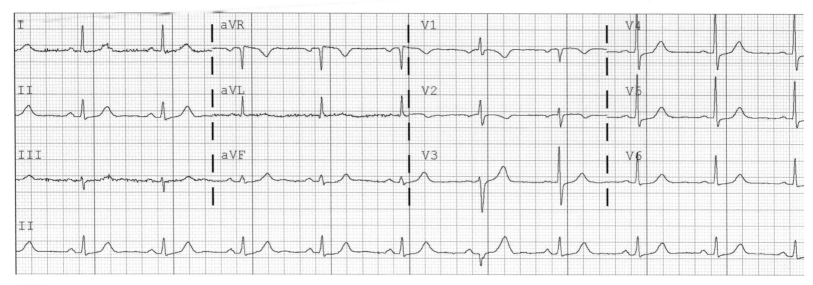

ECG 35.2

EXPLANATION

STEMI This is a left main ST-segment elevation myocardial infarction (STEMI)—perhaps the mother of all STEMIs! These patients are extremely critical and prompt action must be taken.

There are diagnostic ST elevations in leads I, aVL, and V_2 to V_5, including aVR.

By the time the patient was brought to the catheterization laboratory, the patient had developed cardiogenic shock and respiratory failure from acute congestive heart failure. The patient was intubated and venous–arterial extracorporeal membrane oxygenation (VA-ECMO) was placed for optimal hemodynamic support.

Being able to recognize this acute ECG pattern could lead to timely notification of backup services such as cardiothoracic surgery and the ECMO team.

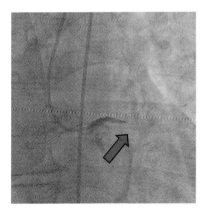 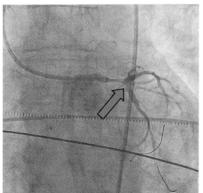 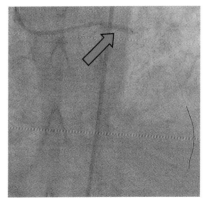 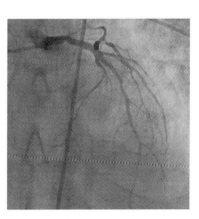

Figure 35.1   Figure 35.2   Figure 35.3   Figure 35.4

Left main occlusion (Figure 35.1, *red arrow*). Angioplasty (Figure 35.2 and 35.3, *blue arrow*). Final angiogram (Figure 35.4) showing restored flow through the left main into the left anterior descending coronary artery (LAD) and left circumflex coronary artery (LCx).

Case 36

PRESENTATION

A 59-year-old non-English-speaking female with hypertension and dyslipidemia presents after several days of chest pain. The pattern of her pain was classic for angina. She had been using non-Western medical therapies for these symptoms. Her symptoms, however, did not improve and she presented to the emergency department.

▸▸ **Presenting Electrocardiogram: Would You Activate the Cath Lab?**

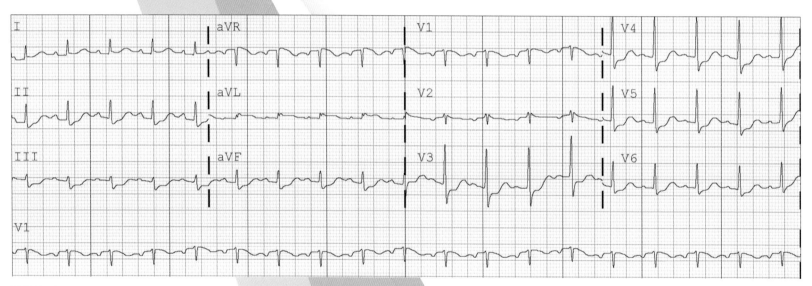

ECG 36.1

There is no prior electrocardiogram (ECG) available for comparison, a repeat ECG was performed (see ECG 36.2).

▶▶ Repeat Electrocardiogram: Would You Activate the Cath Lab?

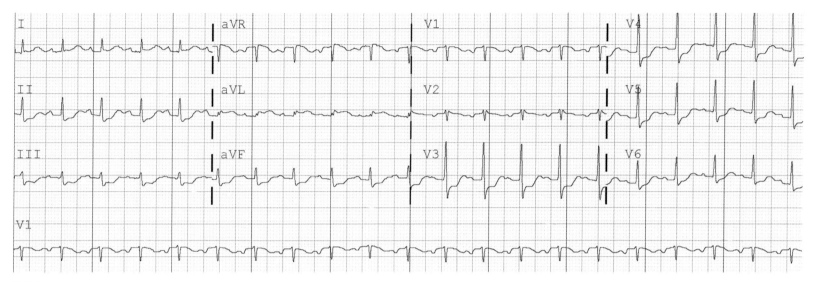

ECG 36.2

EXPLANATION

STEMI The ECG demonstrates sinus tachycardia with an isolated 1-mm ST elevation in lead aVL, but notably a horizontal ST depression with tall R in lead V_3. There are horizontal ST depressions in the inferior/lateral leads as well. In the appropriate clinical context, as in this one, posterior myocardial infarction (MI) should be considered.

Left circumflex coronary artery (LCx) lesions are notorious for being "electrically silent" and can be easily misclassified as a non–ST-segment elevation myocardial infarction (NSTEMI), which does not warrant emergent catheterization. This patient had an isolated posterior MI with only horizontal ST depression with tall R in lead V_3 to demonstrate it. The submillimeter ST elevation in lead I and ST depression in the inferolateral leads also heightens the concern for acute myocardial ischemia. In such a scenario, consider a posterior lead ECG (leads V_7 to V_9). Review Case 4.

The borderline abnormal ECG combined with the language barrier led to a delay in cardiac catheterization by 2 days. The catheterization showed a mid-LCx 95% to 99% culprit lesion, which matches with the findings of posterior infarction on ECG. Ad hoc angioplasty was not performed due to concerns about compliance with dual antiplatelet therapy.

Angioplasty and stenting were eventually scheduled to address the LCx lesion. Unfortunately, the patient succumbed to a ventricular free wall rupture while awaiting for the procedure. The patient had a dismal clinical course despite a surgical patch repair.

Risk factors for free wall rupture include advanced age, female gender, first MI, anterior wall MI, ST elevation or Q-wave development on the initial ECG, a large infarct size, and a late or failed angioplasty.[1]

Reference

1. Nakatani D, Sato H, Kinjo K, et al.; Osaka Acute Coronary Insufficiency Study Group. Effect of successful late reperfusion by primary coronary angioplasty on mechanical complications of acute myocardial infarction. *Am J Cardiol.* 2003;92(7):785-788.

Case 37

PRESENTATION

A 69-year-old male non-English-speaking male with hypertension, dyslipidemia, and former tobacco use presents with acute-onset chest pain while swimming. He could not continue with his exercise routine and was visibly short of breath.

▶▶ **Presenting Electrocardiogram: Would You Activate the Cath Lab?**

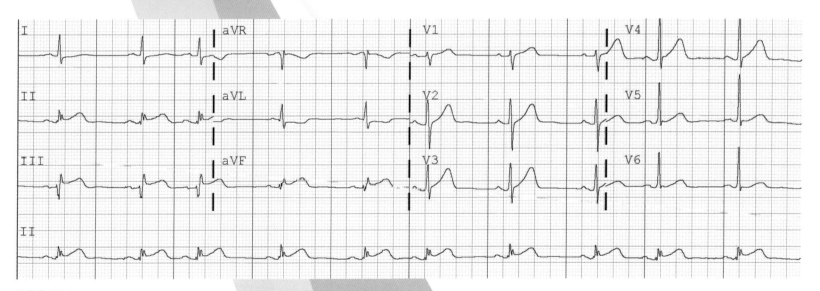

ECG 37.1

There is no prior electrocardiogram (ECG) available for comparison.

EXPLANATION

 STEMI   The ECG shows a straightforward 1-mm ST elevation in leads III and aVF consistent with acute inferior infarction.

However, on emergent catheterization, the culprit vessel was the proximal left anterior descending coronary artery (LAD)!

Why were there **inferior** *leads involved in this* **anterior** *ST-segment elevation myocardial infarction (STEMI)?*

On angiogram, the patient was found to have patent small nondominant RCA and left circumflex coronary arteries (LCx). Anatomically, this patient's LAD compensated by "wrapping-around" left ventricular apex to supply the inferior wall. Hence, with the acute proximal LAD disease, the inferior wall became most ischemic and therefore the most pronounced on the ECG.

The patient had a "wraparound LAD" that supplies not only the anterior/anterolateral myocardium, but also the inferior aspect of the left ventricle (LV; *blue arrow*); see Figure 37.1. An acute lesion in the proximal portion of the large LAD vessel (*red arrow*) caused watershed ischemia to the inferior portion of the LV and cause inferior ST elevations (rather than the "expected" anterior/anterolateral ST elevations typical for LAD lesions) on the presenting ECG. **Anatomic variations can affect the accuracy of localizing the culprit vessel based on the ECG alone.**

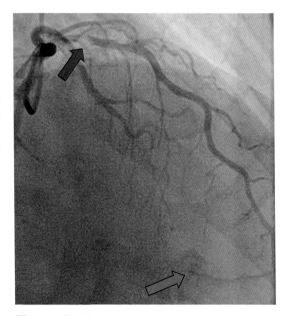

Figure 37.1

Case 38

PRESENTATION

The patient from Case 37 complains of vague 3 out of 10 chest discomfort 3 days after successful drug-eluting stent placement to the proximal left anterior descending coronary artery (LAD).

His vital signs were stable. The discomfort was intermittent without associated symptoms of shortness of breath.

▶▶ **Presenting Electrocardiogram: Would You Activate the Cath Lab?**

Electrocardiogram (ECG) obtained 3 days post-successful proximal LAD stenting for ST-segment elevation myocardial infarction (STEMI).

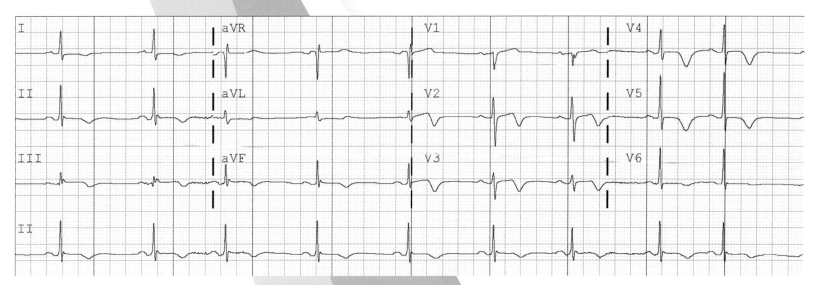

ECG 38.1

EXPLANATION

⌐⊏MI   The follow-up ECG shows biphasic ST changes that would typically be concerning for anterior ischemia. However, these anterior ST-T segment changes are manifestation of evolving changes post–myocardial infarction (MI) and not from acute vessel (or stent) closure.

It is important to recognize the evolving ST-T segment changes that can be expected after MI, with and without coronary revascularization. Clearly, with successful and timely coronary revascularization, the natural history of ST-T segment changes from an MI can be altered. For example, the development of permanent Q waves can be minimized.

In light of the patient's perceived discomfort post-MI, causes such as post-MI pericarditis and other mechanical/structural complications, including papillary muscle rupture, free wall/septal wall rupture, and infarct expansion, need to be considered. Note that acute stent thrombosis, yet another possible complication post-angioplasty, would typically present with clear-cut ST elevations (ie, convex tombstones), which are not present on the patient's follow-up ECG.

Evolving ECG changes during an MI.

Prompt coronary revascularization (ie, short ischemic time) may yield complete and immediate resolution of ST elevations and minimize the formation of Q waves. **However, subsequent post-revascularization ECGs may still demonstrate a period of evolving T-wave inversions in the leads that were affected by the infarction; the T-wave changes will eventually normalize (Figure 38.1).**

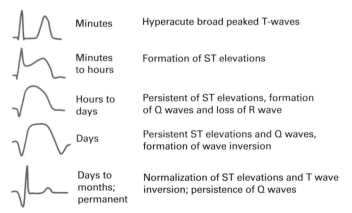

Minutes — Hyperacute broad peaked T-waves

Minutes to hours — Formation of ST elevations

Hours to days — Persistent of ST elevations, formation of Q waves and loss of R wave

Days — Persistent ST elevations and Q waves, formation of wave inversion

Days to months; permanent — Normalization of ST elevations and T wave inversion; persistence of Q waves

Figure 38.1

ECG 1 month later (ECG 38.2).

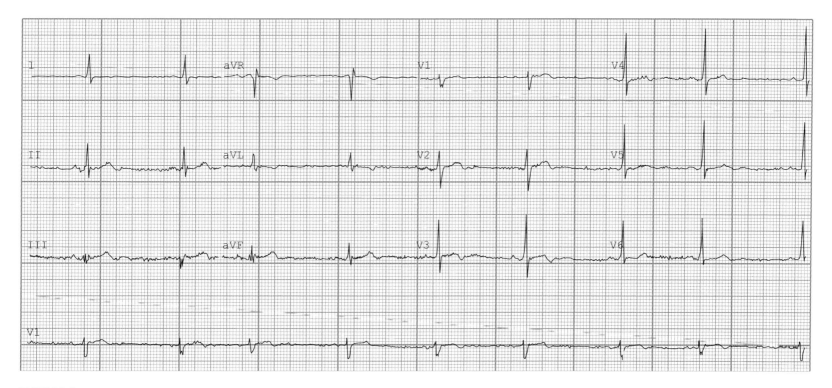

ECG 38.2

Note the evolving T-wave changes 1 month later—the anterior biphasic T-wave changes are still present, while the inferior T-wave changes have largely resolved.

ECG 5 months later (ECG 38.3).

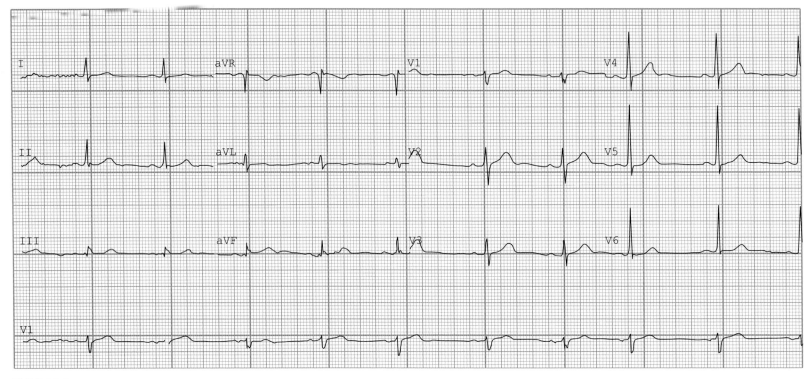

ECG 38.3

ST-T changes have all normalized; there are no pathologic Q waves noted with the prompt coronary revascularization.

Case 39

PRESENTATION

A 49-year-old physician presents with acute-onset substernal "crushing" chest pain. He is diaphoretic, short of breath, and very anxious appearing on examination.

▶▶ **Presenting Electrocardiogram: Would You Activate the Cath Lab?**

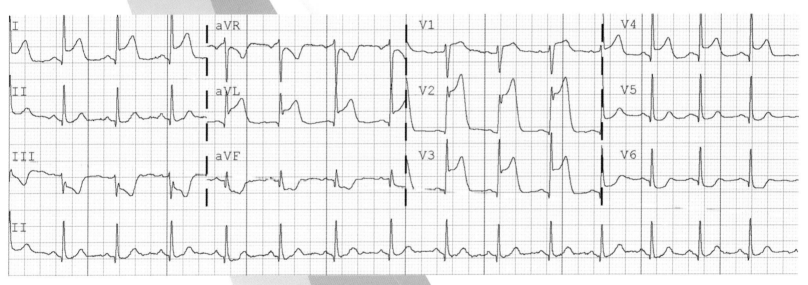

ECG 39.1

There is no prior electrocardiogram (ECG) available for comparison.

EXPLANATION

STEMI   Anterior–lateral ST elevations of acute infarction.

Emergent catheterization revealed proximal left anterior descending coronary artery (LAD) culprit lesion. The patient was treated (ie, "door-to-balloon time") within 90 minutes of arrival to the hospital. The symptom-to-balloon (ie, "ischemic time") was less than 2 hours.

ECG post–percutaneous coronary intervention (PCI) was performed; see ECG 39.2.

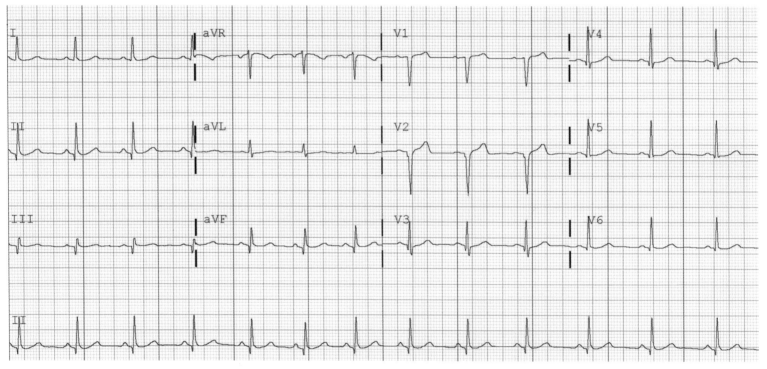

ECG 39.2

Note the resolution of anterolateral ST elevations post-emergent PCI of the proximal LAD lesion.

Case 40

PRESENTATION

Forty-eight hours after the patient from Case 39 suffers from anterior ST-segment elevation myocardial infarction (STEMI), the in-house physicians are prompted to obtain an electrocardiogram (ECG), as the patient reports slight 2 out of 10 vague chest discomfort. Mild shortness of breath was reported. Overall, the symptoms he is describing are much milder than his symptoms on the day of initial presentation.

▸▸ **Presenting Electrocardiogram: Would You Activate the Cath Lab?**

ECG was obtained 2 days post-successful proximal left anterior descending (LAD) stenting for STEMI.

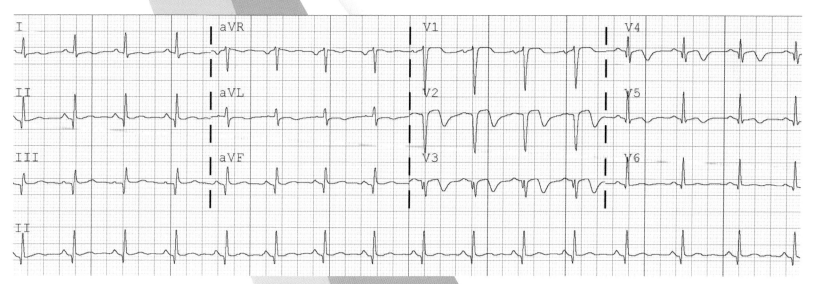

ECG 40.1

EXPLANATION

FCMI   Just as in Case 38, the patient's ST changes are reflective of the naturally occurring ST-segment changes post–myocardial infarction (MI), even after successful and timely revascularization.

Generally speaking, prompt revascularization as in this case, would lead to immediate and dramatic improvement in the ST-segment elevation. However, a period of biphasic ST changes with T-wave inversion may still occur in the leads that were initially affected by the acute ischemia. In cases of LAD infarction, these evolving ST-T-wave changes can be dramatic enough to appear worrisome. Review Case 38.

Serum creatine kinase (CK) remained down-trending, and repeat echocardiogram did not demonstrate any new findings.

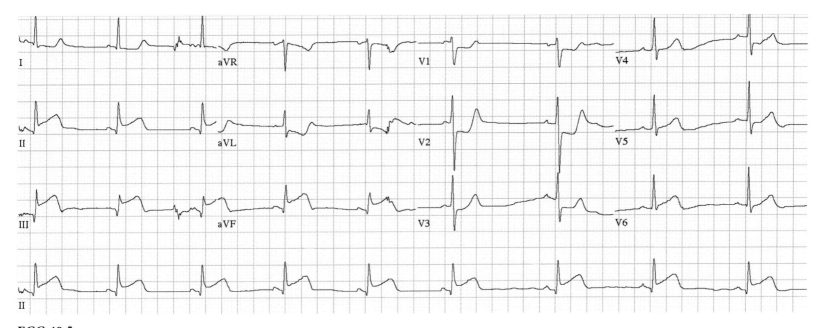

ECG 40.2

ECG 40.2 is from a patient who sustained a large proximal right coronary artery (RCA) infarction, who was promptly revascularized soon after his chest pain started. The next ECG shows the immediate post-MI ECG (see ECG 40.3).

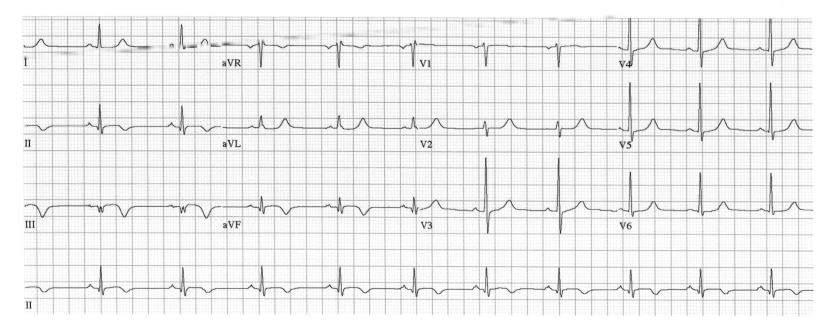

ECG 40.3

Note the immediate resolution of the inferior ST elevations. However, note the evolving ST-T changes on the inferior leads on an ECG performed 1 day after (see ECG 40.4).

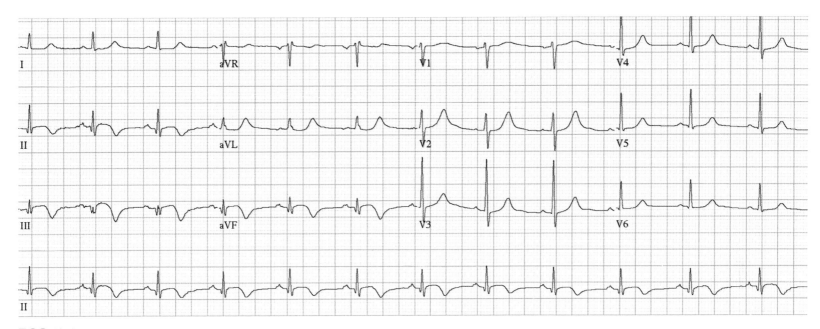

ECG 40.4

Vague chest discomfort with the ECG changes mentioned previously prompted a repeat catheterization. The angiogram not surprisingly demonstrated patent RCA stent and no new coronary disease. The inferior ST changes are reflective of the "expected" evolving ST changes that can be seen post-MI. Stent thrombosis (or acute closure of the stent) would typically yield the similar ST changes as seen on the initial STEMI ECG.

Case 41

PRESENTATION

A 58-year-old female with history of migraine and hypertension was found by her family to be unresponsive at home. The family reports headaches for the past 1 day and was not aware of any prior cardiac history.

She was intubated in the field and was brought to the hospital.

▶▶ **Presenting Electrocardiogram: Would You Activate the Cath Lab?**

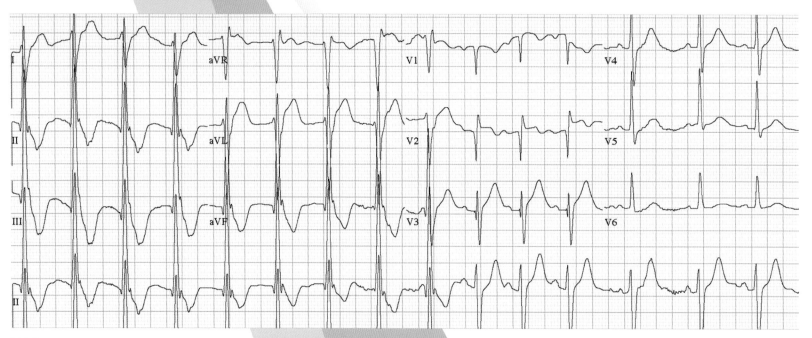

ECG 41.1

There is no prior electrocardiogram (ECG) available for comparison.

EXPLANATION

FEMI The ECG demonstrates sinus rhythm and marked QT-interval prolongation. Deep T-wave inversion is seen in the inferior leads, and ST elevations in leads V_2, V_3, and aVL concerning for acute anterior/lateral territory infarction.

Despite the ischemic-appearing ECG changes, this was a case of a large intracranial hemorrhage. Acute rise in intracranial pressure from larges strokes, bleeds, and acutely enlarging brain masses can cause dramatic changes on ECG. Findings can include marked T-wave changes (also termed "cerebral T waves") with prolonged QT intervals, bradycardia (Cushing reflex: triad of hypertension, bradycardia, and irregular respiration), and ST-T changes that can mimic acute coronary ischemia.

It is believed that cardiac dysfunction (whether be on basis on ECG changes, elevated serum troponin levels, or myocardial dysfunction on echocardiogram) in association with intracranial hemorrhage is neurally mediated and does not reflect an acute coronary syndrome.[1]

On initial presentation, the ECG gave support toward a diagnosis of myocardial ischemia. Conceivably, ischemia could have led to malignant arrhythmias and potentially caused the patient's collapse. Fortunately, in this case, a computed tomography (CT) head was also performed, which diagnosed the large intracranial hemorrhage. The catheterization was aborted and instead, the patient was transferred to a Neurosurgery Center. Such case comes as a reminder to the clinical presentation of ST elevations that are not from acute coronary ischemia.

Reference

1. Okabe T, Kanzaria M, Rincon F, Kraft WK. Cardiovascular protection to improve clinical outcomes after subarachnoid hemorrhage: is there a proven role? *Neurocrit Care.* 2013;18(2):271-284.

Case 42

PRESENTATION

A 53-year-old male with human immunodeficiency virus (HIV) and hypertension presents with 2 episodes of syncope. The patient reports having intermittent prolonged episodes of substernal chest pain for the past week, along with occasional lightheadedness and dizziness.

On arrival to the emergency department, he was hypotensive and bradycardic.

▸▸ **Presenting Electrocardiogram: Would You Activate the Cath Lab?**

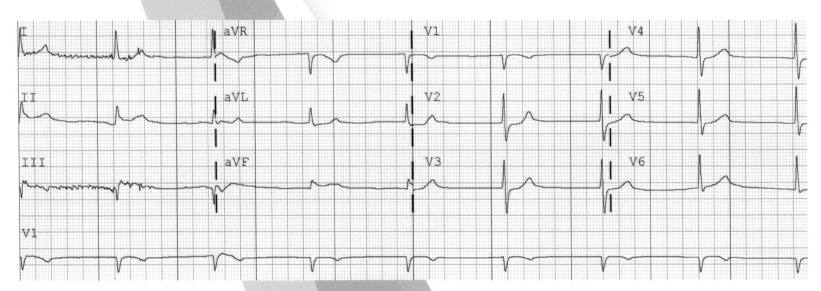

ECG 42.1

There is no prior electrocardiogram (ECG) available for comparison.

EXPLANATION

STEMI   The ECG demonstrates sinus arrest with junctional escape rhythm. There is 1-mm ST elevation in leads III and aVF consistent with acute inferior infarction; the tall R wave with ST depression in lead V$_2$ suggests associated posterior infarction.

Angiogram revealed occlusion of **nondominant** right coronary artery (**RCA**).

The importance of the nondominant RCA can be overlooked, especially given title "nondominant." But as illustrated in this case, the patient had experienced hypotension and sinus arrest with bradycardic junctional rhythm from the acute coronary syndrome of this nondominant vessel. Subsequent echocardiogram also revealed decreased right ventricular (RV) function.

Vessel "dominance" is merely an anatomic definition. The vessel that gives rise to the posterior descending artery (PDA) is termed the "dominant" vessel. It is believed that approximately 70% of people are right dominant, 10% are left dominant (the PDA branch arises from the left circumflex coronary artery [LCx]), and 20% are codominant (the PDA branches arises from both the RCA and LCx) (Figures 42.1 to 42.3).[1]

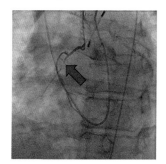 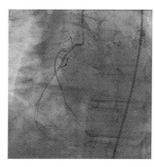

Figure 42.1   **Figure 42.2**   **Figure 42.3**

The culprit lesion is noted in a nondominant mid-RCA (*red arrow*), treated with angioplasty and stenting (*blue arrow*). Despite its apparent diminutive size, this vessel infarct was enough to cause hemodynamic disruption with RV dysfunction and junctional rhythm.

Reference

1.   Fuster V, Alexander RW, O'Rourke RA. *Hurst's the heart.* 10th ed. New York, NY: McGraw-Hill; 2001: 53.

Case 43

PRESENTATION

A 48-year-old female presents with acute onset of acute 10 out of 10 chest pain. She reports a history of coronary artery disease (CAD) with previous drug-eluting stent (DES) placement to the right coronary artery (RCA) greater than 5 years ago and is an active tobacco user.

She states that she has been compliant with her medications, but reports that her physicians instructed her to stop clopidogrel 2 weeks ago. She continued taking aspirin daily.

▶▶ **Presenting Electrocardiogram: Would You Activate the Cath Lab?**

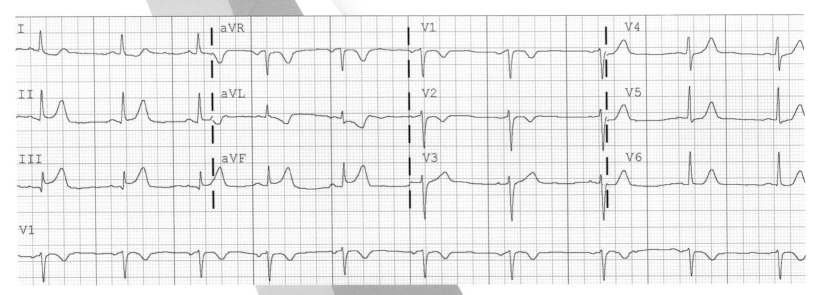

ECG 43.1

A prior electrocardiogram (ECG) is available for comparison (see ECG 43.2).

▶▶ Prior Electrocardiogram for Comparison

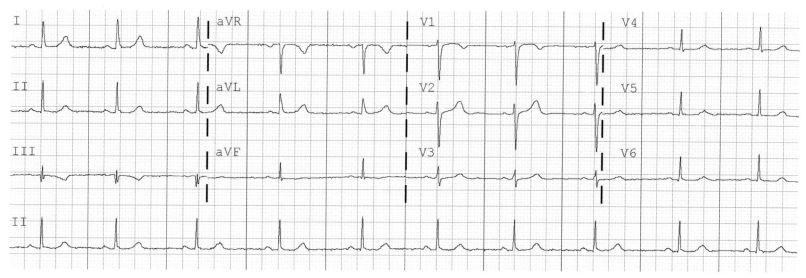

ECG 43.2

EXPLANATION

 3TEMI The ECG demonstrates inferior ST-segment elevation myocardial infarction (STEMI).

The patient had a very late stent thrombosis of her RCA DES placed greater than 5 years ago. Stent thrombosis should still be a consideration even many years post-DES implantation. Delayed vascular healing, stent malapposition, and neoatherosclerosis are some possible mechanisms.[1] In addition, the temporal relationship between the cessation of clopidogrel and stent thrombosis in this patient raises the possibility of aspirin resistance.[2]

References

1. Kaliyadan A, Siu H, Fischman DL, et al. "Very" very late stent thrombosis: acute myocardial infarction from drug-eluting stent thrombosis more than 5 years after implantation. *J Invasive Cardiol.* 2014;26(9):413-416.
2. Gori AM, Marcucci R, Migliorini A, et al. Incidence and clinical impact of dual nonresponsiveness to aspirin and clopidogrel in patients with drug-eluting stents. *J Am Coll Cardiol.* 2008;52(9):734-739.

Case 44

PRESENTATION

A 31-year-old male with a history of aortic and mitral valve replacement after prior endocarditis presents with profound dyspnea. The patient had been nauseated and had vomiting for the past week. Although he does not report chest pain, he mentions his breathing is labored with even minimal exertion and appears lethargic.

In the emergency department, the patient is hypotensive and an electrocardiogram (ECG) was performed.

▶▶ **Presenting Electrocardiogram: Would You Activate the Cath Lab?**

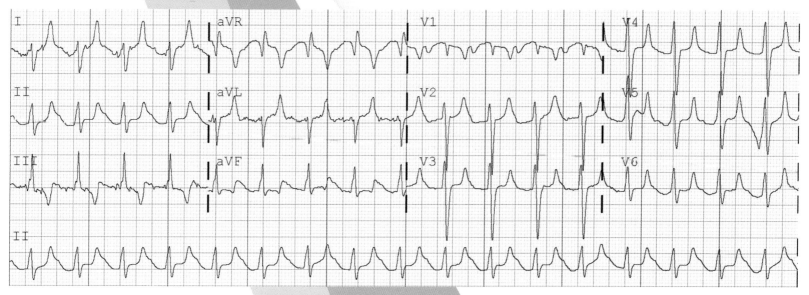

ECG 44.1

There is no prior ECG available for comparison.

EXPLANATION

 ECG The ECG demonstrates sinus tachycardia with first-degree atrioventricular (AV) block and tall, narrow, and peaked T waves diffusely.

Peaked T waves may appear not only as an early sign of an acute myocardial ischemia, but also as a consequence of metabolic derangement including hyperkalemia. Indeed, this is a case of hyperkalemia and not acute coronary syndrome. The patient in the clinical scenario turned out to have multiorgan failure in setting of septic shock. The patient had acute renal and liver dysfunction, and as a result, the patient's serum potassium was 7.3 mmol/L (*normal range is 3.5 to 5.0 mmol/L*).

The determination of "peaked T waves" can be a subjective one. Without a previous ECG for comparison, it is often difficult to objectively determine if a T wave is "peaked," "tall," "narrow," "tented," or "broad"—adjectives commonly used to describe abnormal T-wave morphology in setting of various degrees of hyperkalemia.

There are no formal ranges for what is considered mild, moderate, and severe hyperkalemia and not every patient manifests a predictable pattern of ECG changes with incremental rise in serum potassium levels. In general, early mild/moderate hyperkalemia is associated with narrow, tall, peaked T waves; referred to as T-wave "tenting." With this stage of narrow, tall, and peaked T waves, the ST segment can often be flat (as seen in leads V_2, V_3, V_5, and V_6). As hyperkalemia becomes very severe, the QRS can appear stretched out and the T waves can be broad and bizarre appearing.

In comparison, peaked T waves of myocardial ischemia are described as broad and the ST segment is not flat. The patient's presentation with 1 week of illness and ST changes on ECG were not consistent with acute ischemia. Performing urgent cardiac catheterization in this patient including exposure of contrast agents in setting of renal failure may be more harm than good. After hydration, treatment of sepsis, and normalization of the potassium, the ECG changes resolved (see ECG 44.2).

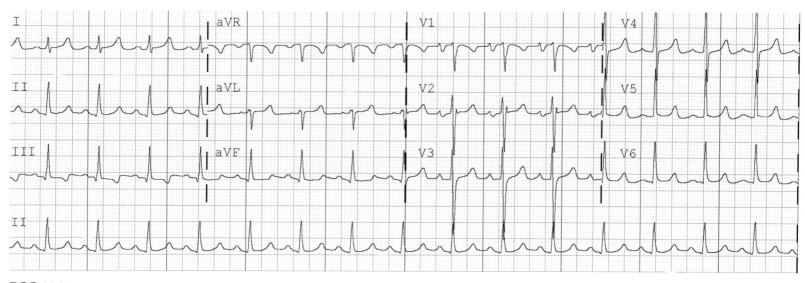

ECG 44.2

Repeat ECG with normal range serum potassium.

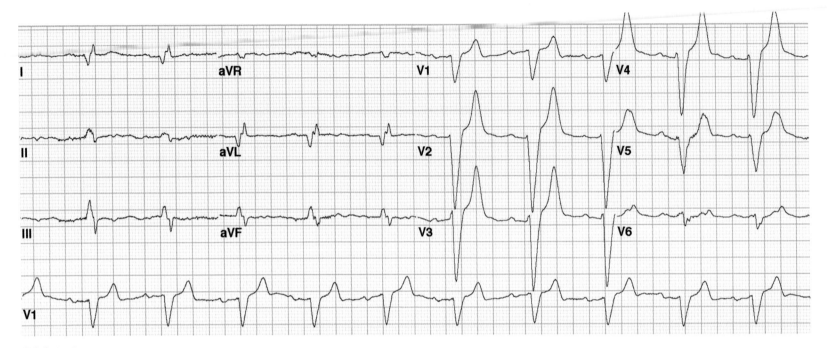

ECG 44.3

This is an ECG of a patient who has a history of noncompliance with hemodialysis regimen who presents with volume overload and hyperkalemia. ECG demonstrates new findings of first-degree AV block with bizarre appearing wide complex QRS complexes consistent with an intraventricular conduction delay (IVCD). The T waves appear broad and peaked compared with his previous ECG; the patient's serum potassium was 8.7 mmol/L (*normal range is 3.5 to 5.0 mmol/L*. Emergent hemodialysis was performed and an ECG was repeated; see ECG 44.4.

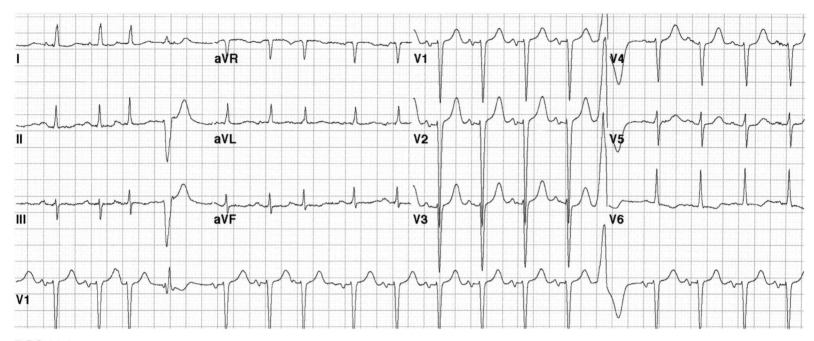

ECG 44.4

ECG 44.4 was obtained shortly after emergent dialysis. The ECG showed return of his baseline
ST-T pattern with resolution of the widened QRS and peaked T waves.

Case 45

PRESENTATION

A 37-year-old male with poorly controlled hypertension and a history of noncardiac chest pain presents to the emergency department with recurrent chest pain. His chest pain has both typical and atypical features, which acutely worsens in the morning, prompting him to seek medical attention.

▸▸ **Presenting Electrocardiogram: Would You Activate the Cath Lab?**

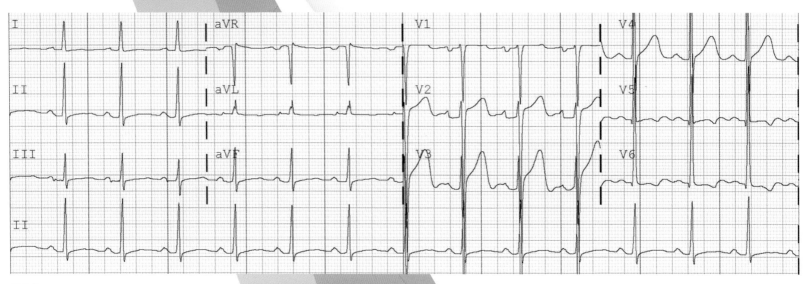

ECG 45.1

A prior electrocardiogram (ECG) is available for comparison (see ECG 45.2).

▶▶ Prior Electrocardiogram for Comparison

ECG 45.2 is an ECG from 2 years ago.

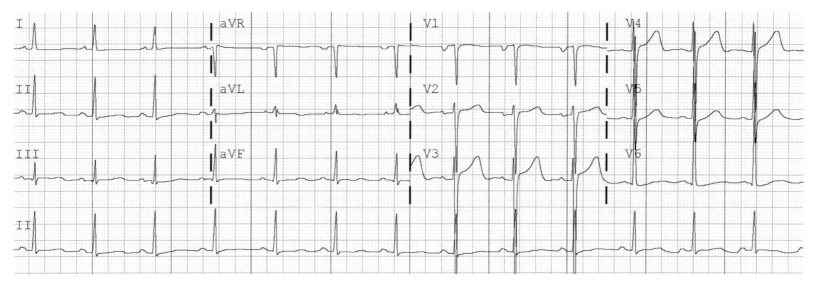

ECG 45.2

Another prior ECG is available for comparison; see ECG 45.3.

▶▶ Prior Electrocardiogram for Comparison

ECG 45.3 is an ECG from 5 years ago

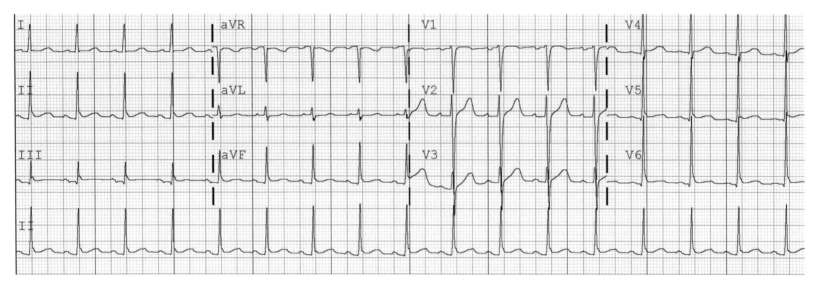

ECG 45.3

EXPLANATION

FEMI   The ECG demonstrates sinus rhythm, left atrial enlargement, left ventricular hypertrophy (LVH) with secondary repolarization, and ≥2-mm ST elevation in leads V_2 and V_3. This should raise the consideration of anterior ischemia.

After review of the patient's symptoms and cardiac risk factors, the patient was indeed taken for urgent catheterization and fortunately had normal coronary arteries.

LVH often limits the certainty of diagnosis for acute coronary ischemia. There are proposed criteria to help distinguish ischemia in setting of LVH; however, all met with limitations regarding diagnostic accuracy.[1] In this example, if applying the methodology from the paper by Armstrong et al, the presenting ECG would not suggest ischemia. The amplitude of ST elevation divided by the RS wave in leads V_1, V_2, or V_3 is <25%; acute ischemia is therefore unlikely.[2]

Sometimes without frank contraindications, proceeding with coronary angiography is the safest and quickest means to manage the patient. Review Cases 16, 18, 19, and 20.

The ST elevations on the presenting ECG reflect repolarization changes of LVH. Note that the QRS voltage, as well as the repolarization pattern in LVH, can change over time.[3] Occasionally, these changes may be as a result of lead placement. Interestingly, in this patient, the voltage amplitude increase correlates with the gradual increase in left ventricular (LV) mass index (via echocardiogram parameters) over a 5-year period likely due to poorly controlled hypertension. **Temporal changes in cardiac structure may render a baseline ECG difficult to use as comparison.**

References

1. Brady WJ, Chan TC, Pollack M. Electrocardiographic manifestations: patterns that confound the EKG diagnosis of acute myocardial infarction-left bundle branch block, ventricular paced rhythm, and left ventricular hypertrophy. *J Emerg Med.* 2000;18(1):71-78.
2. Armstrong EJ, Kulkarni AR, Bhave PD, et al. Electrocardiographic criteria for ST-elevation myocardial infarction in patients with left ventricular hypertrophy. *Am J Cardiol.* 2012;110(7):977-983.
3. Birnbaum Y, Alam M. LVH and the diagnosis of STEMI—how should we apply the current guidelines? *J Electrocardiol.* 2014;47(5):655-660.

Case 46

PRESENTATION

A 61-year-old female with well-controlled type 1 diabetes on insulin, hypertension, and dyslipidemia presents with acute retrosternal 10 out of 10 chest and abdominal pain. She appeared unwell, weak, and had diaphoresis.

Initial workup was consistent with mild diabetic ketoacidosis (DKA), with an anion gap and a serum glucose of more than 400 mg/dL. Her initial serum troponin was negative.

▶▶ **Presenting Electrocardiogram: Would You Activate the Cath Lab?**

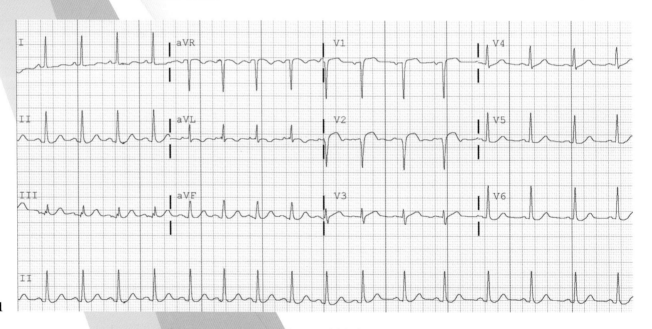

ECG 46.1

A prior electrocardiogram (ECG) is available for comparison (see ECG 46.2).

▶▶ Prior Electrocardiogram for Comparison

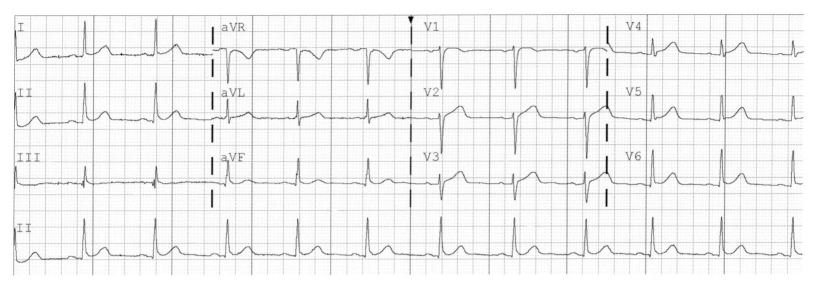

ECG 46.2

EXPLANATION

STEMI   There is 1-mm ST elevation in lead V_1 with >2-mm ST elevation in lead V_2, consistent with anteroseptal infarction, with reciprocal ischemic ST segments in diffuse leads. In comparison to a prior ECG, these ischemic changes are new.

Initially, with the reassuring negative first troponin, the patient was managed for DKA. Cardiology was urgently consulted when the second set of troponins were markedly elevated and noted the ECG changes. This case serves as a reminder to consider acute myocardial infarction (MI) as a potential stressor leading to DKA. The pathophysiology involves the increased demands of insulin in setting of the acute stress of the MI, when the failing pancreas is unable to provide the insulin. This leads to rise in blood glucose, causing dehydration and additional stress; the vicious cycle of DKA ensues.[1]

The patient was found to have a culprit 99% mid-left anterior descending coronary artery (LAD) lesion on urgent cardiac catheterization. Noteworthy is that patients with severe DKA may preclude proceeding with catheterization due to severe acidosis, renal impairment, and poor mental status. In addition, serum hyperkalemia may be present (despite a total body depletion of potassium) and can lead to misleading ST-segment changes that can be mistaken for MI.[2] Review Case 44.

References

1. Delaney MF, Zisman A, Kettyle WM. Diabetic ketoacidosis and hyperglycemic hyperosmolar nonketotic syndrome. *Endocrinol Metab Clin North Am.* 2000;29(4):683-705, V.
2. Moulik PK, Nethaji C, Khaleeli AA. Misleading electrocardiographic results in patient with hyperkalemia and diabetic ketoacidosis. *BMJ.* 2002;325(7376):1346-1347.

Case 47

PRESENTATION

A 57-year-old female with hypertension, dyslipidemia, and diabetes presents with unrelenting 10 out of 10 retrosternal chest pain. The patient is clutching her chest, and reports occasional discomfort that radiates to her back and jaw. She is diaphoretic and in apparent physical distress.

▸▸ **Presenting Electrocardiogram: Would You Activate the Cath Lab?**

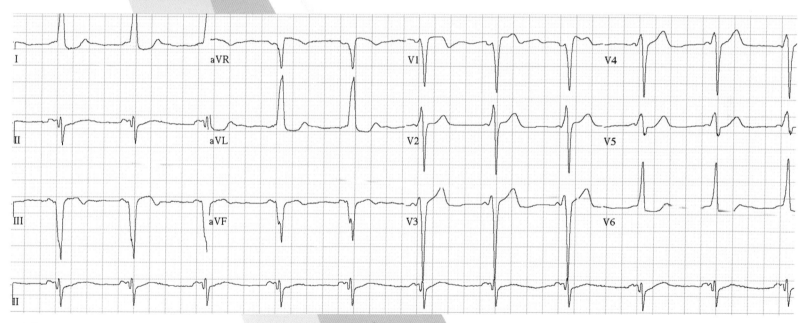

ECG 47.1

There is no prior electrocardiogram (ECG) available for comparison.

EXPLANATION

FEMI The ECG demonstrates sinus rhythm, 1-mm ST elevation in lead III and 1-mm ST elevation in V_1 concerning for inferior/right ventricular (RV) ischemia; there were diffuse ST depressions in the lateral leads.

The patient was taken for urgent cardiac catheterization. The coronary arteries were normal, but angiography revealed that the patient had a type A aortic dissection! As there was difficulty during the coronary angiogram in passing the pigtail catheter through the ascending aorta, this prompted an angiogram of the aortic root ("aortogram"). The ascending aortogram demonstrated a linear flap outlined by the contrast concerning for a type A aortic dissection. A subsequent emergent computed tomography (CT) scan confirmed the diagnosis and revealed the extent of dissection propagation. The patient was sent for emergency thoracic surgery.

Remember to consider noncardiac etiologies of chest pain, namely potentially life-threatening diseases, such as aortopathies and pulmonary embolism, when acute obstructive coronary atherosclerosis has been excluded. ST changes on presenting ECG likely reflect intermittent episodes of coronary flow obstruction by the highly mobile intimal flap of the aortic wall.

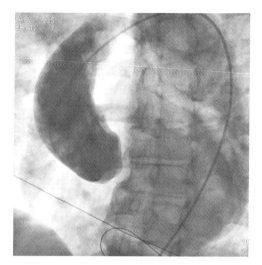

Figure 47.1

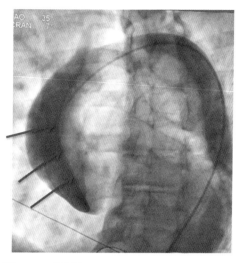

Figure 47.2

Figures 47.1 and 47.2. On ascending aortography, a type A aortic dissection flap can be appreciated; the *red arrows* point to the moving intimal flap of the dissection.

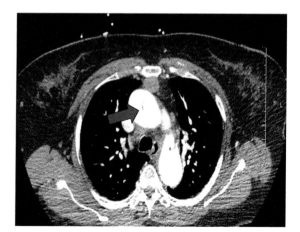

Figure 47.3

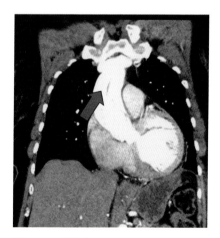

Figure 47.4

Figures 47.3 and 47.4. Type A dissection confirmed on CT chest with intravenous contrast; the *red arrows* point to the dissection flap in the ascending aorta.

Case 48

PRESENTATION

A 51-year-old female was having a heated argument with family members. Suddenly, she developed sharp back pain, with shortness of breath and diaphoresis. She came immediately to the emergency department for evaluation. She denies any previous cardiac problems. Chest x-ray was clear without a widened mediastinum. Aside from hypertension, other vital signs were stable.

▸▸ **Presenting Electrocardiogram: Would You Activate the Cath Lab?**

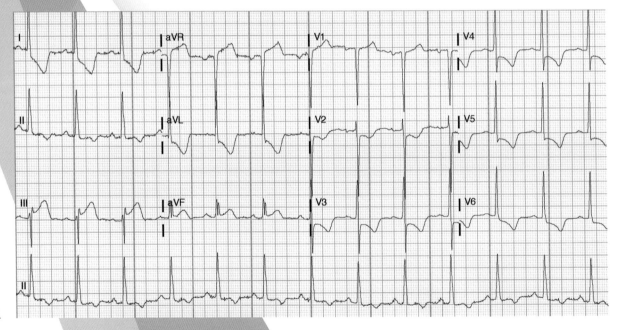

ECG 48.1

There is no prior electrocardiogram (ECG) available for comparison.

EXPLANATION

STEMI   The ECG demonstrates sinus rhythm, left ventricular hypertrophy (LVH) with secondary repolarization, and inferior ST elevations consistent with acute inferior ST-segment elevation myocardial infarction (STEMI).

However, angiography revealed that the mid-right coronary artery (RCA) 100% occlusion was caused by a Type A dissection. **This is a true nightmare for an interventional cardiologist.** This patient was emergently transferred to a center with computed tomography (CT) surgery capability.

Myocardial ischemia may accompany Type A aortic dissections in roughly 1% to 2% of cases, and affects the RCA more than the left coronary system. There are several mechanisms for how Type A dissections can cause myocardial infarction:

1) the intimal flap from the aortic wall becomes large enough that it prolapses into the vessel lumen during diastole ("intussusception"),
2) direct antegrade extension of the flap from the aorta into the coronary artery,
3) circumferential detachment and hematoma formation of the dissection causing external compression of the coronary vessel.[1]

This diagnosis is potentially catastrophic and its importance should be noted. Although this is a relatively rare scenario, cases like these remind us to never let our guard down. Review Case 47.

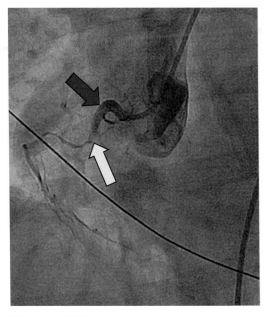

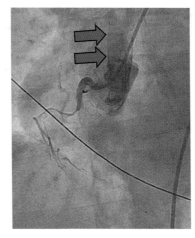

Figure 48.2

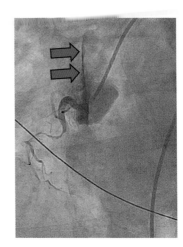

Figure 48.3

Note the dissection flap in the RCA (*red arrow*, pointing to a linear white streak within the RCA indicating dissection) extending from the aorta leading to a mid-RCA occlusion (*yellow arrow*). The intimal flap in the ascending aorta is indicated in the *blue arrows*, indicative of a Type A dissection.

Figure 48.1

Deciphering which patient has a "simple" STEMI versus an aortic dissection with a concomitant STEMI can be difficult, especially with the constraints of the demanding "90-minute door-to-balloon time." Nevertheless, the 2010 American College of Cardiology/American Heart Association (ACC/AHA) guidelines recommends a low threshold for suspicion for acute aortic disease in patients having the following several features:

Presentation: chest, back, or abdominal pain; syncope, and ischemia of nervous, cardiac, mesenteric, or peripheral artery systems.

Underlying conditions: Marfan syndrome, connective tissue disease, genetic aortopathy syndromes.

High-risk pain features: chest, back, or abdominal pain described as abrupt in intensity and a tearing/sharp/stabbing quality.

High-risk physical examination findings: perfusion deficits (ie, pulse differential between left and right sides, focal neurologic changes), aortic regurgitation murmur, or hypotension/shock.[2]

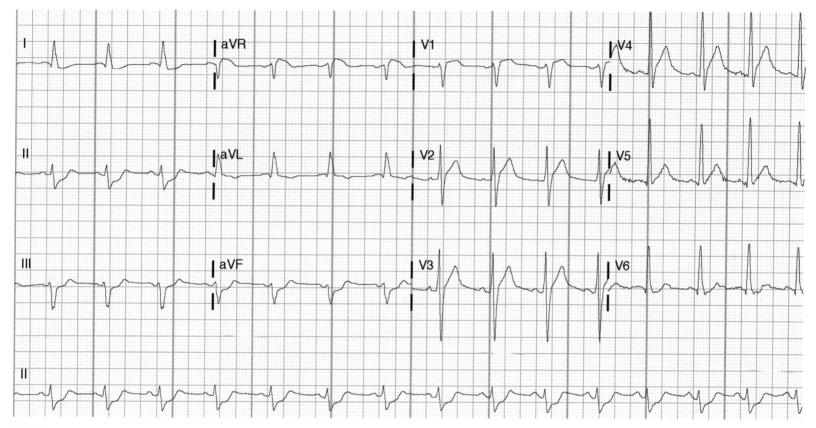

ECG 48.2

ECG 48.2 is of another example of a patient with an acute Type A dissection with an abnormal ECG showing anterior ST elevations with reciprocal ST depressions. This is a case of a 64-year-old male with hypertension. He reported severe acute unrelenting upper back and chest pain, and had a syncopal episode. A cardiac catheterization team was activated when this ECG was noted. However, the symptoms were worrisome enough for the cardiologist to first request a CT scan to rule out aortic pathology. Indeed, the patient had an acute Type A dissection! Unfortunately, the patient developed cardiac arrest shortly after the CT scan was performed and expired.

References

1. Lentini S, Perrotta S. Aortic dissection with concomitant acute myocardial infarction: from diagnosis to management. *J Emerg Trauma Shock.* 2011;4(2):273-278.
2. Hiratzka LF, Bakris GL, Beckman JA, et al.; American College of Cardiology Foundation/American Heart Association Task Force on Practice Guidelines; American Association for Thoracic Surgery; American College of Radiology; American Stroke Association; Society of Cardiovascular Anesthesiologists; Society for Cardiovascular Angiography and Interventions; Society of Interventional Radiology; Society of Thoracic Surgeons; Society for Vascular Medicine. 2010 ACCF/AHA/AATS/ACR/ASA/SCA/SCAI/SIR/STS/SVM Guidelines for the diagnosis and management of patients with thoracic aortic disease. A Report of the American College of Cardiology Foundation/American Heart Association Task Force on Practice Guidelines, American Association for Thoracic Surgery, American College of Radiology, American Stroke Association, Society of Cardiovascular Anesthesiologists, Society for Cardiovascular Angiography and Interventions, Society of Interventional Radiology, Society of Thoracic Surgeons, and Society for Vascular Medicine. *J Am Coll Cardiol.* 2010;55(14):e27-e129.

Case 49

PRESENTATION

A 78-year-old male with a history of coronary artery disease (CAD) and sick sinus syndrome with a dual chamber pacemaker, presents with chest pain. He is status post a recent drug-eluting stent placement to the ramus intermedius for in-stent restenosis and has been compliant with all his cardiovascular medications.

He describes an intense 8 out of 10 chest pain that awoke him from sleep at 2 AM. It radiates to the back. The emergency department performed a computed tomography (CT) scan (which ruled out an aortic dissection) after noting the initial serum troponin was negative. The patient's chest discomfort persisted.

▶▶ **Presenting Electrocardiogram: Would You Activate the Cath Lab?**

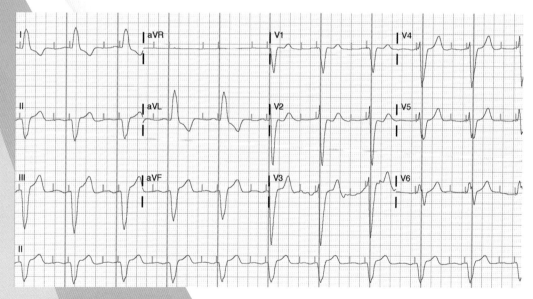

ECG 49.1

A prior electrocardiogram (ECG) is available for comparison (see ECG 49.2).

▶▶ Prior Electrocardiogram for Comparison

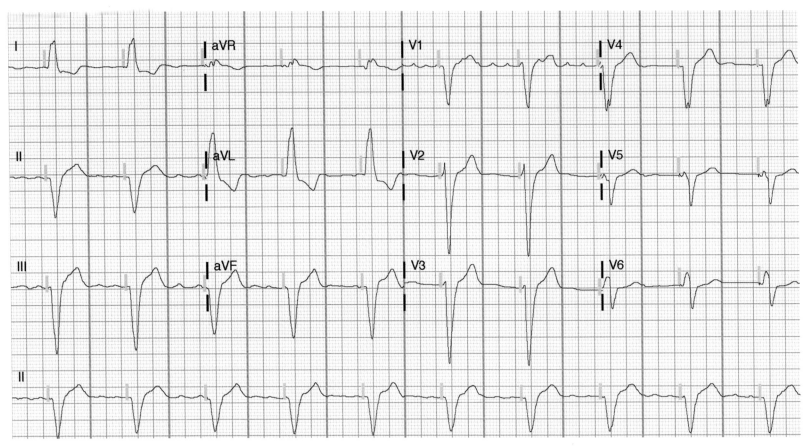

ECG 49.2

EXPLANATION

STEMI   The first ECG demonstrates atrial-sensed ventricular paced rhythm with concordant ST depressions in V_2 (in setting of right ventricle [RV]-paced rhythm) suggestive of acute ischemia.

The typical ventricular pacing (ie, RV pacing, and not biventricular pacing) pattern manifests an ECG that closely resembles a typical left bundle branch block (LBBB). And likewise, ischemia in setting of right ventricular pacing can be detected using the Sgarbossa criteria; review Case 11. Note, however, that the sensitivity is low and may be even lower when Sgarbossa criteria are applied for right ventricular pacing as in this case.[1]

On the presenting ECG, there is concordance in the ST deviation in lead V_2, which is new from the baseline (see next ECG) and is diagnostic for acute coronary ischemia. On catheterization, the patient had an acute stent thrombosis of the ramus intermedius, and another layer of drug-eluting stent was deployed.

Anatomically, the left main typically bifurcates into the left anterior descending coronary artery (LAD) and left circumflex coronary artery (LCx); however, in roughly 10% to 20% of patients, the left main trifurcates into the LAD, ramus intermedius, and the LCx.

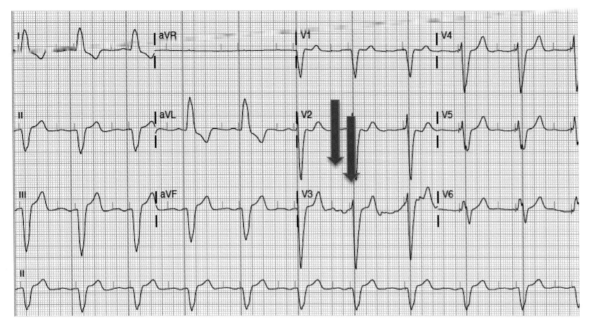

ECG 49.3

Review the presenting ECG and note the ST-J point depression in lead V_2. In normal LBBB and in RV pacing, the ST-J point is elevated when the primary vector of the QRS is negative (ie, normally discordant ST deviation; the *red arrows* should be pointing in opposite direction). However, in this patient with active ischemia, both the ST-J point and primary QRS vector are negative and therefore showing concordance (*red arrows*).

Reference

1. Sgarbossa EB, Pinski SL, Barbagelata A, et al. Electrocardiographic diagnosis of evolving acute myocardial infarction in the presence of left bundle-branch block. GUSTO-1 (Global Utilization of Streptokinase and Tissue Plasminogen Activator for Occluded Coronary Arteries) Investigators. *N Engl J Med.* 1996;334(8):481-487.

Case 50

PRESENTATION

A 60-year-old non-English-speaking male with history of lifelong tobacco use presents with 30 minutes of chest pain while moving furniture. He describes the pain in the "heart and lungs," with a sharp 10 out of 10 in quality.

▶▶ **Presenting Electrocardiogram: Would You Activate the Cath Lab?**

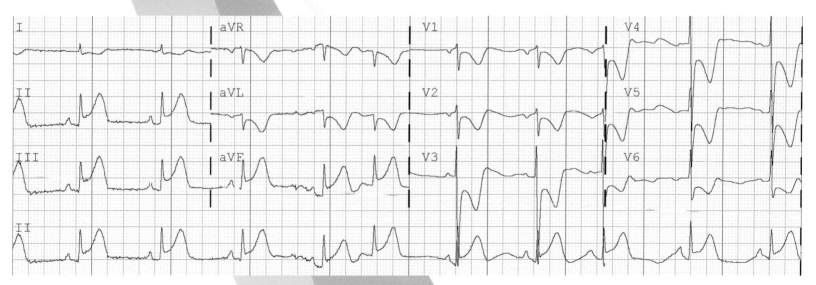

ECG 50.1

There is no prior electrocardiogram (ECG) available for comparison.

EXPLANATION

 STEMI The ECG demonstrates inferior ST elevations, with diffuse ST changes suggestive of global myocardial ischemia.

On emergent coronary angiography, the proximal right coronary artery (RCA) culprit is apparent, *but why the dramatic anterior/lateral ST-T changes?*

The dramatic ST depressions likely reflect severe concomitant high-grade left anterior descending coronary artery (LAD) and diagonal branch vessel disease. The acute stress of the myocardial infarction (MI) with the compensatory hyperdynamic function of the anterior wall, likely led to the ischemic appearing changes in the anterior/lateral leads during the inferior ST-segment elevation myocardial infarction (STEMI). He ultimately underwent coronary artery bypass graft (CABG) for his LAD/diagonal disease after a period of clinical stability.

Signs of multivessel disease in patients who present with an acute coronary syndrome are important to note, because these patients are likely to be "sicker."[1] Review Case 26.

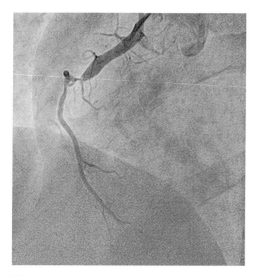

Figure 50.1

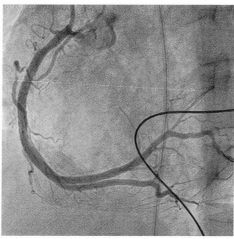

Figure 50.2

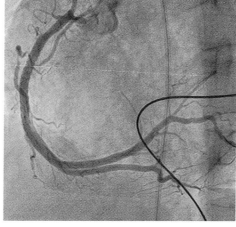

Figure 50.3

Proximal RCA occlusion (*left image*). Final angiogram after RCA angioplasty and stenting (*center image*). Severe diffuse LAD/diagonal branch disease (*blue star; right image*).

Reference

1. Sorajja P, Gersh BJ, Cox DA, et al. Impact of multivessel disease on reperfusion success and clinical outcomes in patients undergoing primary percutaneous coronary intervention for acute myocardial infarction. *Eur Heart J.* 2007;28(14):1709-1716.

Case 51

PRESENTATION

A 37-year-old male, an intravenous drug user, presented with fevers. He was found to have bacteremia and echocardiogram demonstrated aortic valve endocarditis. He was transferred to a tertiary care center for valve surgery.

On arrival to the new hospital, he reported acute onset of dyspnea and chest heaviness. He is diaphoretic and appeared unwell.

▶▶ **Presenting Electrocardiogram: Would You Activate the Cath Lab?**

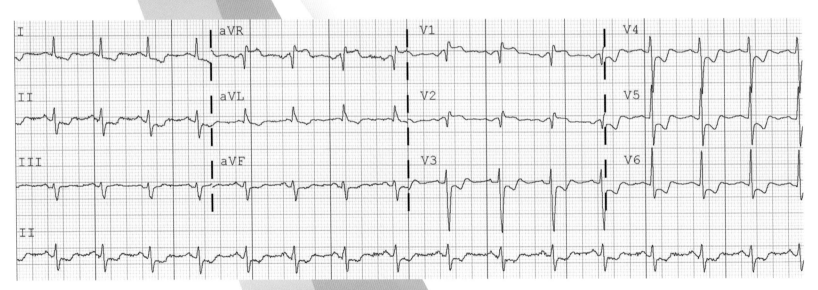

ECG 51.1

A prior electrocardiogram (ECG) is available for comparison (see ECG 51.2).

▶▶ Prior Electrocardiogram for Comparison

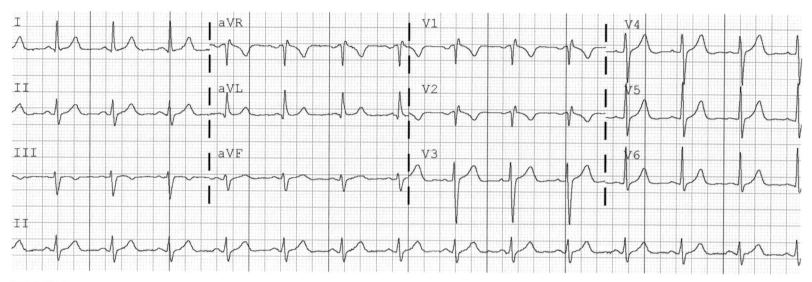

ECG 51.2

EXPLANATION

fEMI The ECG demonstrates sinus rhythm with 1-mm ST elevations in leads V_1 and V_2 (consider anteroseptal injury), along with ST depressions in multiple leads.

This is generally suggestive of global myocardial ischemia; however, this case was not a result of coronary artery occlusion.

Rather, this patient with severe *Staphylococcus aureus* aortic valve endocarditis had developed not only acute severe aortic regurgitation, but also had aortic root abscess. This led to a left ventricular (LV) outflow tract to right ventricular (RV) fistula formation. The ECG changes are a manifestation of acute volume/pressure overload from the aortic regurgitation, hemodynamic changes with the fistula, along with subendocardial ischemia from the hyperdynamic state of severe sepsis.

It is conceivable for septic embolism into the coronary arteries or a clump of bacterial abscess occluding the coronary ostia; however, the ECG changes resolved post emergent surgery (aortic root debridement, fistula patch repair, and aortic valve replacement with a mechanical valve) and the patient did not demonstrate segmental wall motion abnormalities on echocardiogram.

Dramatic ECG changes often prompt one to evaluate for acute coronary artery occlusion; however, this case exemplified the need to keep the overall clinical context in mind, which was endocarditis. A repeat echocardiogram and an expedited cardiothoracic surgery evaluation were the next best step in management in this case.

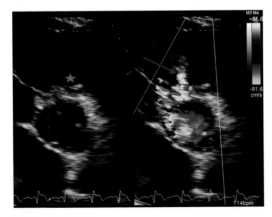

Aortic root abscess (*blue star*) leading to an LV outflow tract to RV fistula (*red arrow*).

Figure 51.1

Case 52

PRESENTATION

A 59-year-old female without previous medical conditions presents with acute prolonged episode of substernal chest pain.

▶▶ **Presenting Electrocardiogram: Would You Activate the Cath Lab?**

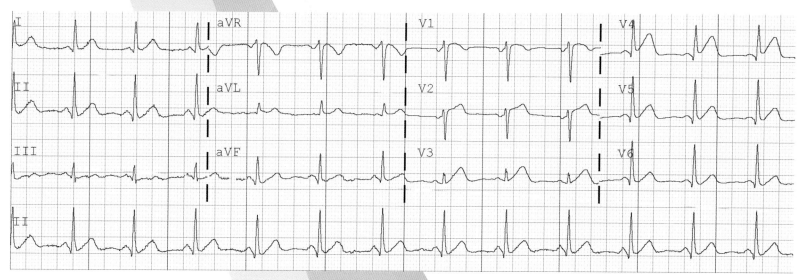

ECG 52.1

There is no prior electrocardiogram (ECG) available for comparison, a repeat ECG was performed (see ECG 52.2).

▶▶ Repeat Electrocardiogram: Would You Activate the Cath Lab?

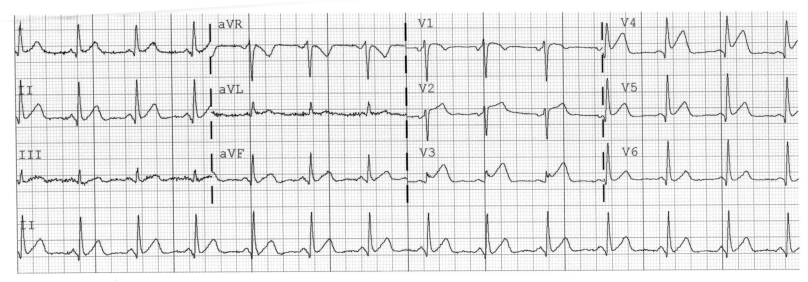

ECG 52.2

EXPLANATION

STEMI   The initial ECG demonstrates 1-mm ST elevation in lead V_1 and 2-mm ST elevation in lead V_2, with broad T waves in leads V_3 to V_6, suggestive of anteroseptal/anterior ischemia.

The initial ECG did in fact meet criteria for acute myocardial infarction (MI); however, these ischemic changes can be subtle. What did not help was the falsely reassuring initial serum troponin that was negative. The repeat ECG was performed after the patient reported recurrence of the substernal chest discomfort. Urgent catheterization would indeed reveal an acute occlusive thrombotic mid-left anterior descending coronary artery (LAD) lesion.

This case showcases the importance of serial ECGs and following through with patient symptoms in the acute setting. ECGs that are subtle or "borderline" of new ischemic changes should be repeated to assure stability.[1]

Reference

1. O'Gara PT, Kushner FG, Ascheim DD et al. 2013 ACCF/AHA guideline for the management of ST-elevation myocardial infarction: executive summary: a report of the American College of Cardiology Foundation/American Heart Association Task Force on Practice Guidelines. *J Am Coll Cardiol.* 2013;61(4):485-510.

Case 53

PRESENTATION

A 46-year-old male visiting from another town and with a reported history of a "stent" placement 3 weeks ago, presents with acute shortness of breath along with sharp/crushing pain that radiated to the left arm and back. This chest tightness lasted several minutes; however, exertional dyspnea remains the prominent symptom.

He admits to intravenous drug and cocaine use. He denied fevers or chills.

▶▶ **Presenting Electrocardiogram: Would You Activate the Cath Lab?**

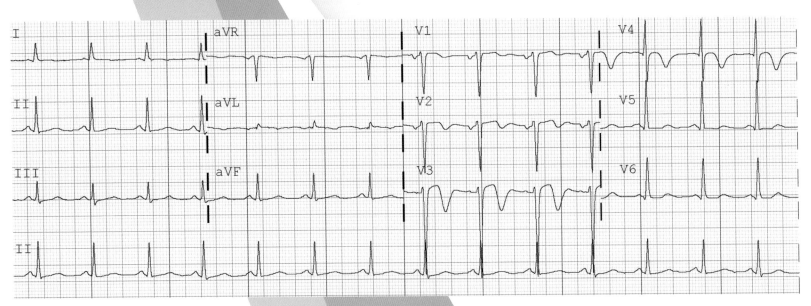

ECG 53.1

There is no prior electrocardiogram (ECG) available for comparison.

EXPLANATION

FEMI   The ECG demonstrates borderline ST elevations in leads V_2 and V_3, with deep T-wave inversions with poor R-wave progression, concerning for anterior ischemia.

The patient's symptoms, recent cardiac history, and marked ST changes made the decision for urgent catheterization unavoidable.

However, the coronaries were patent and there were no stents visualized despite reported by the patient. After obtaining previous medical records, it became apparent that the ECG abnormalities were a manifestation of evolving ST changes (age-indeterminate anterior infarction) from the acute coronary syndrome 3 weeks ago at another hospital (review Cases 3, 38, and 40). At that previous hospitalization, the patient had a mid-left anterior descending coronary artery (LAD) lesion treated with **balloon angioplasty only without stenting** due to concerns for dual antiplatelet therapy compliance, which is required for post-stent placement.

Regarding his symptoms of shortness of breath, the patient was later discovered to have acute severe aortic insufficiency from aortic valve endocarditis, which were new findings when compared to an echocardiogram report obtained from his previous hospitalization. Blood cultures had returned positive for Streptococcus and the patient ultimately required valve replacement. Obtaining collateral information and evaluating for possible alternative etiologies for chest pain symptoms (after the unremarkable cardiac catheterization) were important aspects to this case.

Case 54

PRESENTATION

An 89-year-old male with hypertension and prior stroke presents with sudden onset left-sided chest pain. It came on during exertion, and is associated with shortness of breath but not diaphoresis.

▸▸ **Presenting Electrocardiogram: Would You Activate the Cath Lab?**

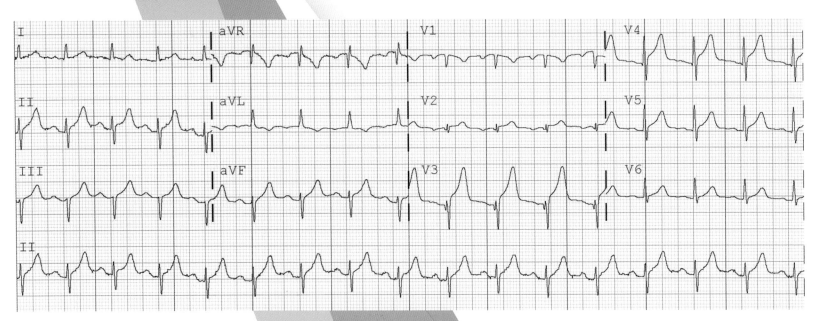

ECG 54.1

A prior electrocardiogram (ECG) is available for comparison (see ECG 54.2).

▶▶ **Prior Electrocardiogram for Comparison**

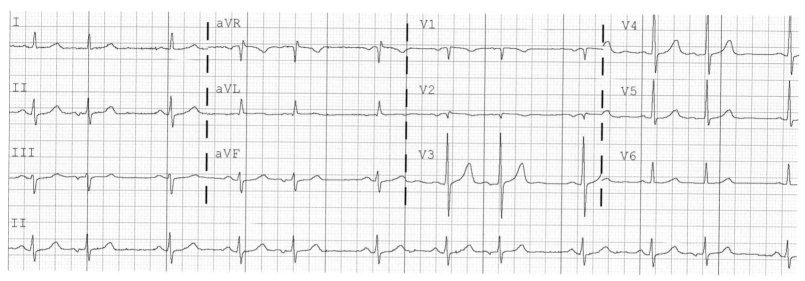

ECG 54.2

EXPLANATION

 STEMI   The ECG demonstrates sinus tachycardia with broad hyperacute T waves, poor R-wave progression, and ST elevations in leads V_3 to V_6 consistent with anterior infarction. The patient had an acute left anterior descending coronary artery (LAD) lesion.

On ECG 54.1, note the fractionated or fragmented QRS complexes best seen in leads V_2 and V_3. Fragmented QRS defined as presence of an additional R wave (R′) or notching in the nadir of the S wave, or the presence of >1 R′ in 2 contiguous leads, corresponding to a major coronary artery territory. This finding has been associated with abnormal electrical conduction through myocardium that is diseased from ischemia and/or fibrosis.[1]

Hyperacute T waves of ischemia are often "broad" with upsloping ST segment. In comparison, T waves of hyperkalemia are often the narrow, peaked, "tented," and with flat ST segment; review Case 44.

Reference

1.   Pietrasik G, Zareba W. QRS fragmentation: diagnostic and prognostic significance. *Cardiol J.* 2012;19(2):114-121.

Case 55

PRESENTATION

A 65-year-old male with dyslipidemia and diabetes presents with intermittent chest pressure for 2 weeks. Occasionally, these episodes might be triggered by exertion or deep inspiration. He denies recent illnesses or fevers.

He went to his primary care physician who obtained an electrocardiogram (ECG).

▶▶ **Presenting Electrocardiogram: Would You Activate the Cath Lab?**

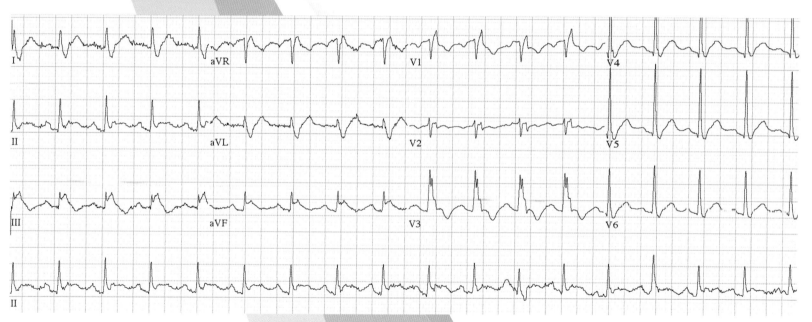

ECG 55.1

There is no prior ECG available for comparison.

EXPLANATION

FFMI   The ECG demonstrates sinus tachycardia, right bundle branch block (RBBB) with ST elevations in leads II, III, and aVF concerning for acute inferior infarction. However, as there is also diffuse PR depression, PR elevation in lead aVR, and borderline diffuse ST elevations, one should also consider pericarditis.

Urgent cardiac catheterization was requested, and the patient had a nonobstructive coronary artery disease (CAD). The patient's clinical presentation seemed inconsistent with an acute coronary syndrome (ie, ST-segment elevation myocardial infarction [STEMI]), especially in light of the duration and quality of symptoms (pleuritic chest pain). As the patient had CAD risk factors, it was reasonable to recommend proceeding with coronary angiogram to exclude concomitant acute CAD, in absence of frank contraindications.

The patient was ultimately discharged from the hospital with a diagnosis of pericarditis and responded well to a course of nonsteroidal anti-inflammatory agents and colchicine treatment.

Case 56

PRESENTATION

A 51-year-old female with previous left anterior descending coronary artery (LAD) stent and active tobacco use and alcohol abuse presents to the emergency department after sustaining a fall while intoxicated. She has multiple left rib fractures and is admitted to the hospital for pain control.

While in the hospital, the patient continues to report left-sided chest pain. Chest x-ray was negative for pneumothorax, and an electrocardiogram (ECG) was performed.

▶▶ **Presenting Electrocardiogram: Would You Activate the Cath Lab?**

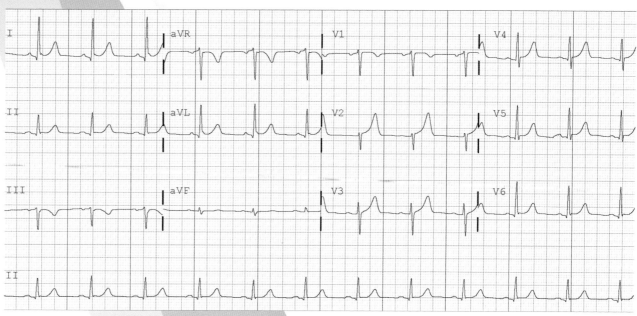

ECG 56.1

There is no prior ECG available for comparison.

The patient continues to report 6 out of 10 chest pain with hypoxia (oxygen saturations in the mid-80%, requiring supplemental oxygen); a repeat ECG was obtained (ECG 56.2).

▶▶ Repeat Electrocardiogram: Would You Activate the Cath Lab?

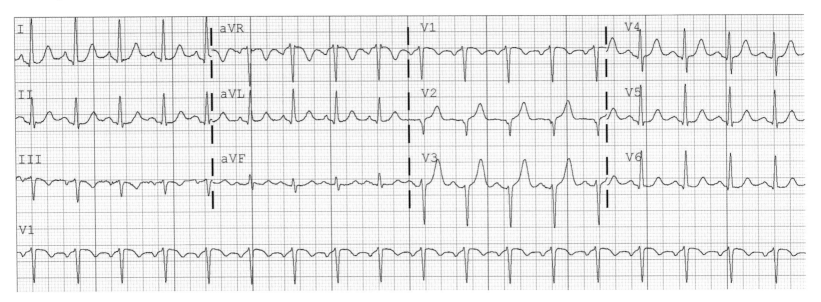

ECG 56.2

After 30 minutes, the patient continues to report chest pain, and has increased to 8 out of 10 in severity. Her serum troponin was negative. *Should further action be taken?*

The two presenting ECGs demonstrated sinus tachycardia, with anteroseptal Q waves, but certainly no obvious ST elevations.

The chest pain could be attributed to the left rib fractures, and the hypoxia could potentially be from splinting and impaired breathing mechanics secondary to the pain.

However, the point of this case is to note the repeat ECG performed approximately 15 minutes later. The patient continues to report increasing left-sided chest pain and that the intravenous (IV) pain medications were ineffective (ECG 56.3).

▶▶ Repeat Electrocardiogram: Would You Activate the Cath Lab?

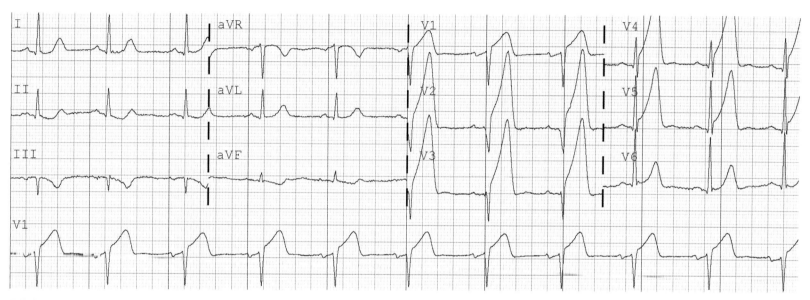

ECG 56.3

EXPLANATION

 STEMI   The last ECG of the series demonstrates broad hyperacute T waves with ST elevations in the anterior leads, consistent with acute infarction.

This case illustrates two key points. The first is that acute coronary syndromes can indeed occur, as the name implies, acutely. Despite two stable ECGs (and also a negative serum troponin), the sudden development of the proximal LAD stent thrombosis coincidentally occurred.

Second, what can never be brought out in a book or in a lecture format are the intangibles of patient care—occasionally, our "gut sense" of a patient's change in clinical status may provoke us to perform yet another diagnostic test, ask the patient yet another question during the patient interview, or go back to the bedside to reexamine the patient. The patient's presentation with left-sided rib fractures certainly complicated the recognition of new superimposing cardiac chest pain. Nevertheless, the escalating patient medication requirement and no history of narcotic dependence had prompted yet another ECG. **Familiarize yourself with the ECG machine in your institution.**

Case 57

PRESENTATION

A 73-year-old male with a pacemaker for history of a "slow heart rate," but no previous known coronary artery disease, presents with intense chest pain while mowing his lawn. On emergency department arrival, he was in obvious distress, but his vital signs were stable.

▸▸ **Presenting Electrocardiogram: Would You Activate the Cath Lab?**

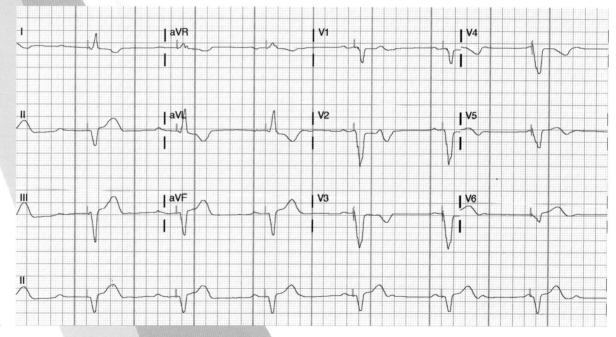

ECG 57.1

There is no prior electrocardiogram (ECG) available for comparison.

EXPLANATION

STEMI   The ECG demonstrates atrial sensed, ventricular-paced rhythm. There is concordance of the ST-J point direction with the primary QRS vector direction, which is abnormal and concerning for myocardial ischemia in setting of right ventricle (RV)-paced rhythm.

Similar to diagnosing ischemia in setting of left bundle branch block (LBBB), the Sgarbossa criteria can be applied to patients with underlying paced rhythm (RV pacing, not biventricular pacing).[1] Review Cases 11 and 49.

Generally, RV-paced beats will demonstrate discordance where the predominant QRS vector and the ST-J deflection are in opposite directions. However, with ischemia, this pattern may be disrupted, and concordance may be present.[1]

The patient had a 100% culprit stenosis of a large left circumflex coronary artery (LCx) artery, which was successfully treated with angioplasty and stenting.

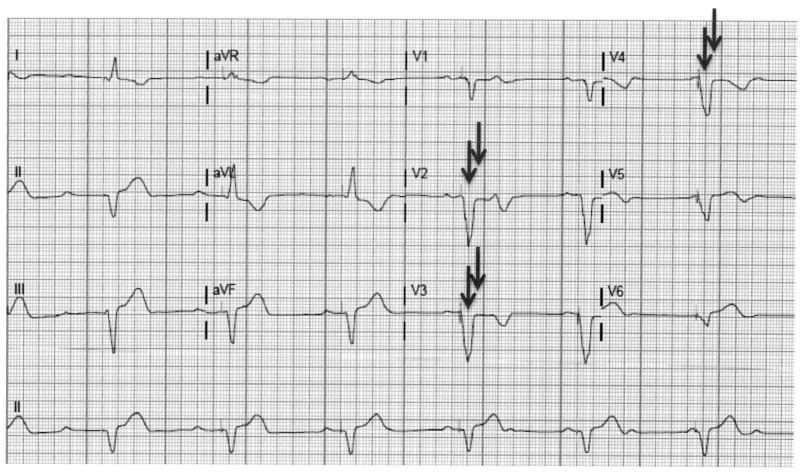

ECG 57.2

Review of the presenting ECG. Note the abnormal concordance of the main QRS vector and the ST-J point, which can be seen in myocardial ischemia (*the red arrows are pointing in the same direction*).

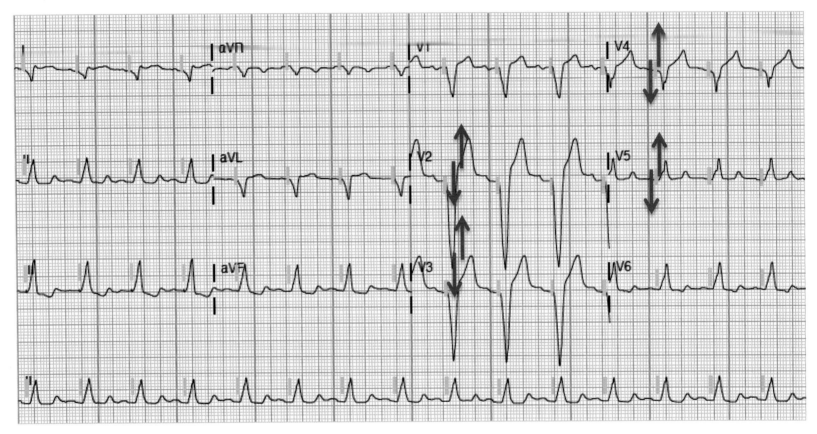

ECG 57.3

Typical RV pacing appears similar to an LBBB, with normal discordance of the main QRS vector and the ST- J point (*red arrows pointing in opposite directions*).

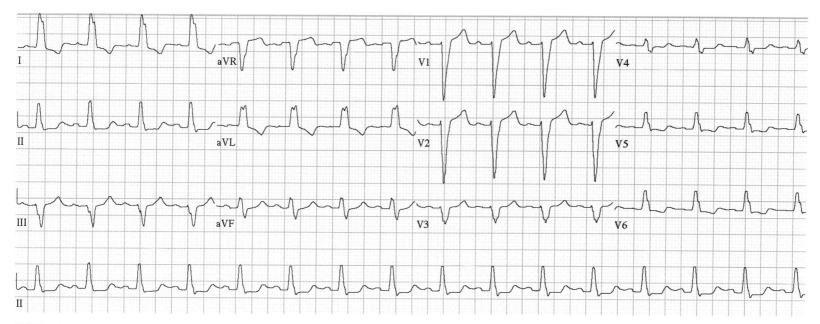

ECG 57.4

ECG 57.4 shows LBBB. Note the similarities with normal RV pacing seen in ECG 57.3.

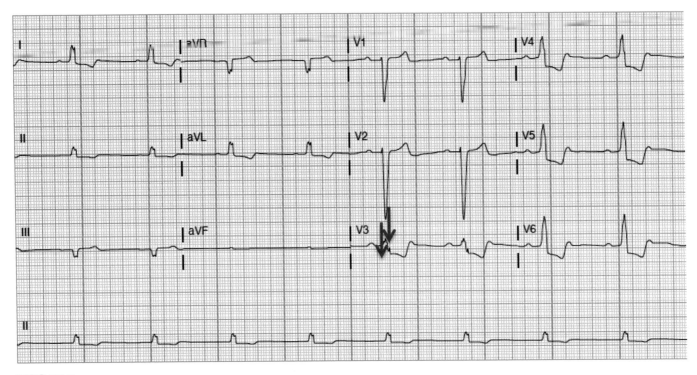

ECG 57.5

This is an example of a patient with acute left anterior descending (LAD) ischemia with baseline LBBB. Note the concordance in lead V₃ (*red arrows*) along with ischemic ST segments in leads V₄ to V₆. Compare this ischemic-LBBB ECG to a nonischemic typical LBBB from ECG 57.4.

Reference

1. Sgarbossa EB, Pinski SL, Barbagelata A, et al. Electrocardiographic diagnosis of evolving acute myocardial infarction in the presence of left bundle-branch block. GUSTO-1 (Global Utilization of Streptokinase and Tissue Plasminogen Activator for Occluded Coronary Arteries) Investigators. *N Engl J Med.* 1996;334(8):481-487.

Case 58

PRESENTATION

A 34-year-old male with poorly controlled hypertension and medication noncompliance presents with retrosternal chest pain while watching television. The pain was persistent, non-radiating and was associated with diaphoresis.

In the emergency department, his blood pressure was persistently elevated at roughly 240s/150s.

▶▶ **Presenting Electrocardiogram: Would You Activate the Cath Lab?**

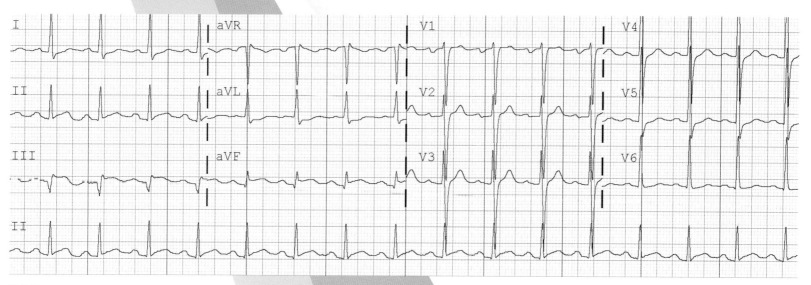

ECG 58.1

There is no prior electrocardiogram (ECG) available for comparison.

EXPLANATION

STEMI   The ECG demonstrates sinus rhythm, left atrial enlargement, left ventricular hypertrophy (LVH), and 1-mm ST elevations in III and aVF concerning for acute inferior ST-segment elevation myocardial infarction (STEMI).

On catheterization, the patient indeed had a distal right posterior descending artery (PDA) occlusion accounting for the presenting ECG. However, several points must be addressed:

1. The right PDA was a small vessel (jeopardizing only a small area of myocardium), and therefore less likely to be of prognostic significance.
2. The blood pressure was markedly elevated (and the concern for increased bleeding risk with full anticoagulation and dual antiplatelet therapy during the percutaneous coronary intervention [PCI]).
3. Concerns with compliance with dual antiplatelet therapy if angioplasty and stenting were to be performed.

Medical therapy without involving angioplasty and stenting was determined to be the next best course of action. Risk factor modification and continued patient education on lifelong medication adherence were emphasized.

Case 59

PRESENTATION

A 72-year-old female with coronary artery disease (CAD) with previous stent placement presents with crescendo pattern of exertional substernal chest pain. Her discomfort increased to the point where chest pain episodes persist for at least 30 minutes.

In the emergency department, she states that she refuses all medical procedures despite presenting to the hospital on her own will. Although she has had previous cardiac stenting procedures, she is fearful to undergo another one.

The patient appears to have full capacity to make all her own medical decisions and has no record of mental illnesses.

▸▸ **Presenting Electrocardiogram: Would You Activate the Cath Lab?**

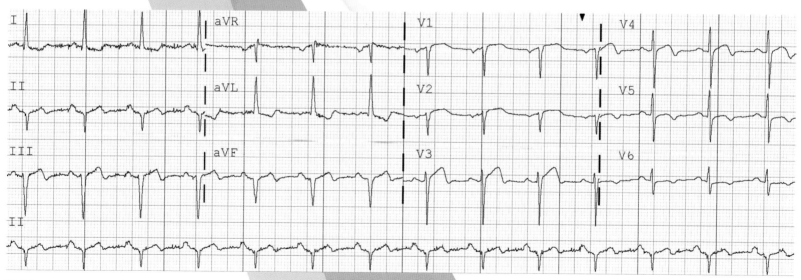

ECG 59.1

A prior electrocardiogram (ECG) is available for comparison (see ECG 59.2).

▶▶ Prior Electrocardiogram for Comparison

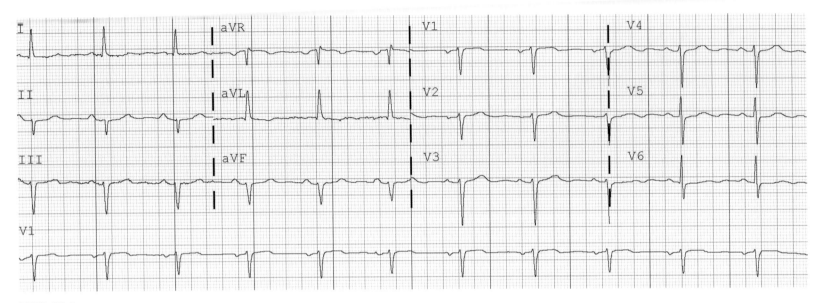

ECG 59.2

EXPLANATION

STEMI   The ECG demonstrates Q waves in the inferior leads suggestive of old infarct and new ST elevations in the anteroseptal/anterior leads concerning for anterior ST-segment elevation myocardial infarction (STEMI).

The curveball to this case was the patient's initial refusal of all medical procedures. **A cardiac catheterization, no matter how emergent, should not be performed without the patient's informed consent, which includes understanding the risk, benefits, alternatives, and rationale**.

While hospitalized, the patient experienced another bout of severe chest pain, and after discussion was finally agreeable for cardiac catheterization. It revealed multivessel disease, with left main 70% stenosis, unstable appearing mid-left anterior descending coronary artery (LAD) 95% stenosis (the culprit lesion), and proximal right coronary artery (RCA) 90% stenosis.

The patient agreed for coronary artery bypass graft (CABG).

Case 60

PRESENTATION

A 56-year-old female with hypertension and known nonobstructive coronary artery disease presents with substernal chest pressure. She mentions that she is undergoing significant emotional distress in light of her father's recent death. The pain has escalated to the point where it now occurs at rest, and is associated with pallor and diaphoresis.

▸▸ **Presenting Electrocardiogram: Would You Activate the Cath Lab?**

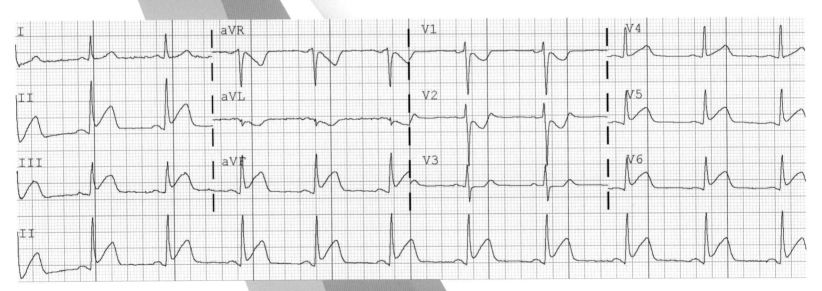

ECG 60.1

There is no prior electrocardiogram (ECG) available for comparison.

EXPLANATION

FEMI   The ECG demonstrates ST elevations consistent with an inferior–posterior–lateral ST-segment elevation myocardial infarction (STEMI). However, the patient's urgent coronary angiogram revealed patent vessels.

This patient had significant wall motion abnormalities on ventriculogram; there was akinesis of the proximal segments of the left ventricle and preservation of the distal wall function. This is in contrast and opposite to the "typical" or "apical" Takotsubo pattern where there is akinesis of the distal segments with preservation of the proximal segments (review Cases 15 and 22). Hence, these cases are referred to as "basal" or "reverse" Takotsubo cardiomyopathy. There are other forms of this transient cardiomyopathy, including "mid-ventricular" and "focal" variants.[1]

The death of the patient's father may have been the stressor, triggering the stress-induced cardiomyopathy with a "reverse" Takotsubo pattern. The patient's wall motion abnormalities and ECG findings resolved in outpatient follow-up several weeks later. Stress-induced cardiomyopathy can cause ST elevations that mimic those caused by coronary ischemia (Figures 60.1 to 60.3).

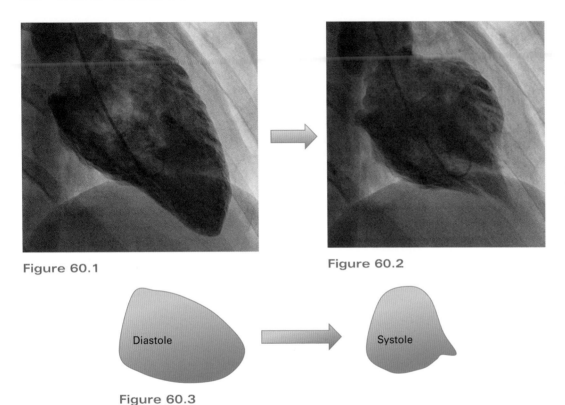

Figure 60.1

Figure 60.2

Figure 60.3

On the patient's ventriculogram, noticed in systole, the basal 1/2 of the ventricle does not contract and actually balloons outward (dyskinetic motion), while the distal 1/2 of the ventricle contracts normally—this is referred to as the "basal" or "reverse" Takotsubo pattern. Review Case 15.

Reference

1. Templin C, Ghadri JR, Diekmann J, et al. Clinical features and outcomes of Takotsubo (stress) cardiomyopathy. *N Engl J Med.* 2015;373(10):929-938.

Case 61

PRESENTATION

A 63-year-old female with type 2 diabetes on insulin, hypertension, and dyslipidemia presents with shortness of breath for the past several days. She had minimal chest pain or pressure.

In the emergency department, she was noted to be hypoxic and tachycardic.

▸▸ **Presenting Electrocardiogram: Would You Activate the Cath Lab?**

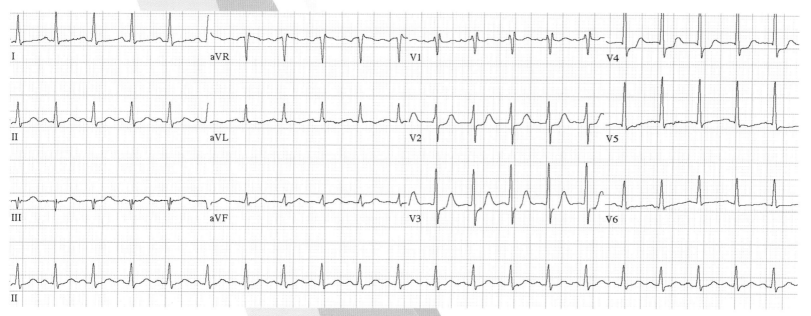

ECG 61.1

There is no prior electrocardiogram (ECG) available for comparison.

EXPLANATION

STEMI The ECG demonstrates sinus tachycardia with anterior ST depressions (ie, leads V$_2$ to V$_4$), concerning for ischemia—in particular, isolated posterior infarction.

The patient's chest symptoms, hypoxia, and tachycardia caused the treating physicians to be concerned for pulmonary embolism; and in this context, they believed the ECG changes to be consistent with "right ventricular strain." The computed tomography (CT) angiogram of the chest was negative for pulmonary embolism, but had findings consistent with congestive heart failure.

After closer inspection of the ECG, it was realized that the anterior ST depressions (ie, horizontal ST depressions in leads V$_2$ to V$_4$ with tall R wave in V$_2$) were actually changes stemming from an isolated posterior wall myocardial infarction. Unfortunately, a posterior lead ECG was not obtained; review Cases 4 and 36. On catheterization, there was acute stenosis of a large OM1 branch likely leading to transient ischemic mitral regurgitation causing "flash" pulmonary edema and hypoxia.

Case 62

PRESENTATION

A 56-year-old male with history of prior coronary artery bypass graft (CABG) presents with sudden onset chest tightness radiating to the bilateral shoulders pain after exertion. The discomfort was persistent and did not resolve with nitroglycerin.

▸▸ **Presenting Electrocardiogram: Would You Activate the Cath Lab?**

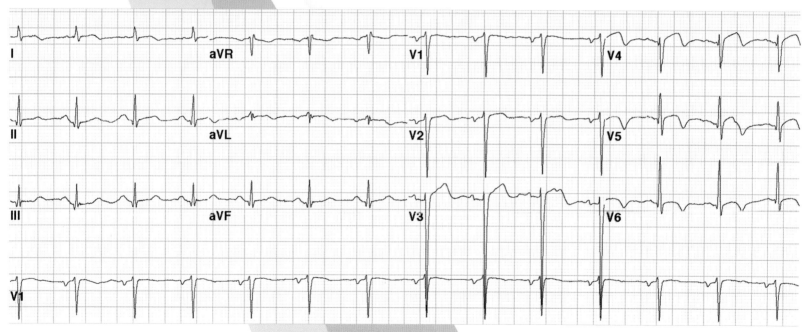

ECG 62.1

A prior electrocardiogram (ECG) is available for comparison (see ECG 62.2).

▶▶ Prior Electrocardiogram for Comparison

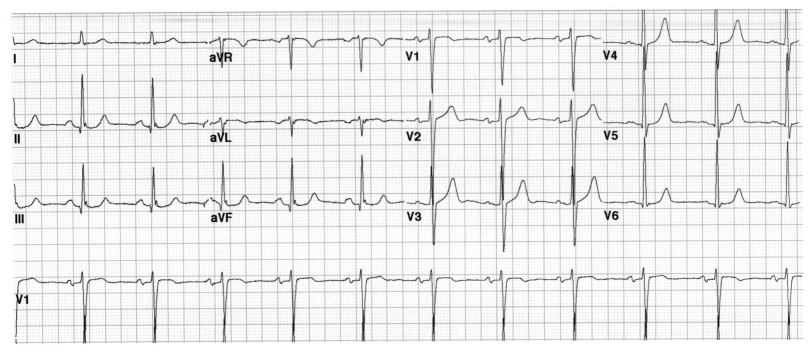

ECG 62.2

EXPLANATION

STEMI   The ECG was diagnostic for anterolateral ST-elevation myocardial infarction.

The patient's bypass anatomy included a sequential left internal mammary artery (LIMA) to the D$_1$ and to the mid-left anterior descending coronary artery (LAD). In an acute setting, isolating the culprit lesion can be challenging in a patient with complex coronary artery anatomy, in particular, patients with prior CABG. Fortunately, the patient had prior angiograms at the institution, which allowed for a baseline angiogram for comparison.

In summary, the native first diagonal was the culprit vessel. The first diagonal also feds the sequential graft that bridges the D$_1$ and the mid/distal LAD; the LIMA graft to the diagonal was known to be occluded. For this patient, the first diagonal serves as an important vessel supplying the anterior and anterolateral segment of the heart, and with an acute lesion in this first diagonal, the anterior–anterolateral territory had become acutely ischemic. See next illustration for details on the coronary anatomy (Figure 62.1).

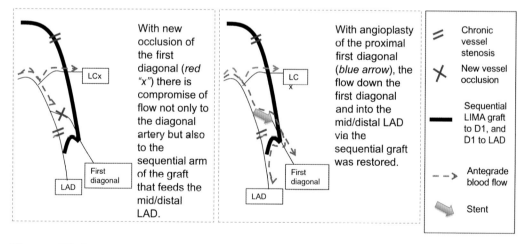

With new occlusion of the first diagonal (red "x") there is compromise of flow not only to the diagonal artery but also to the sequential arm of the graft that feeds the mid/distal LAD.

With angioplasty of the proximal first diagonal (blue arrow), the flow down the first diagonal and into the mid/distal LAD via the sequential graft was restored.

≡ Chronic vessel stenosis

✕ New vessel occlusion

▬ Sequential LIMA graft to D1, and D1 to LAD

--→ Antegrade blood flow

Stent

Figure 62.1

PRESENTATION

A 94-year-old female with hypertension presents to the emergency department with complaints of nagging chest and upper epigastric discomfort and overall lethargy. She appears unwell and in painful distress, but has unremarkable vital signs.

She comes from a senior living facility, who sends a "Do Not Resuscitate/Intubate" document with her. There are no family members present.

▶▶ **Presenting Electrocardiogram: Would You Activate the Cath Lab?**

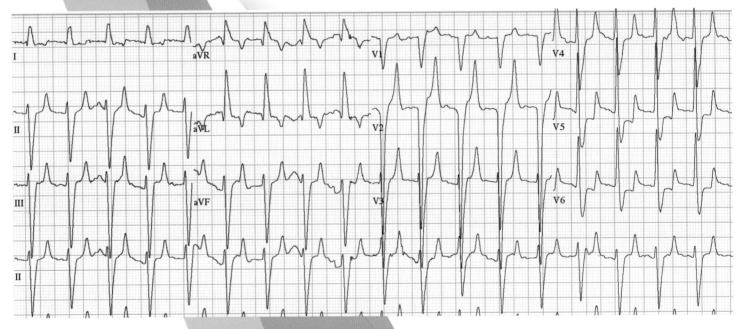

ECG 63.1

A prior electrocardiogram (ECG) is available for comparison (see ECG 63.2).

▶▶ Prior Electrocardiogram for Comparison

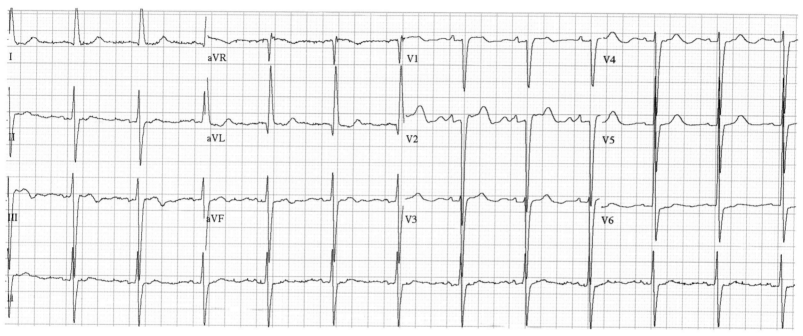

ECG 63.2

EXPLANATION

FFMI   The ECG demonstrates sinus tachycardia with peaked/narrow T waves, prolonged QRS, and anterior ST-J point elevations with lateral ST depressions, which are changes from baseline.

Closer evaluation reveals, however, that the ST contour changes and T-wave morphology are not typical of an acute coronary event. With myocardial infarction, the T waves are generally broad; however, in this patient's ECG, the T waves are pointed and narrow. In addition, the ST segments are occasionally flat (ie, leads II, III, and V_4 to V_6), that is not seen in acute infarction, which would demonstrate elevated/convex ST segment. In the setting of highly atypical chest pain symptoms, the decision was made to wait for the results of the initial laboratory tests and communicate with the family prior to deciding on cardiac catheterization.

The basic metabolic panel returned with a serum potassium level was 9.2 mmol/L (*normal range is 3.5 to 5.0 mmol/L*). The patient turned out to have severe hyperkalemia from acute renal injury secondary to hypovolemia from diuretics, and potassium supplements.

Recognize the subtle differences of ST-T changes that distinguish hyperkalemia and ischemia. The patient received emergent dialysis instead of cardiac catheterization. Review Case 44.

Case 64

PRESENTATION

A 74-year-old female with hypertension, dyslipidemia, active tobacco smoking, and diabetes was brought in to the emergency department by ambulance for acute persistent substernal chest pain. She was detected to have new atrial fibrillation with rapid ventricular response.

▶▶ **Presenting Electrocardiogram: Would You Activate the Cath Lab?**

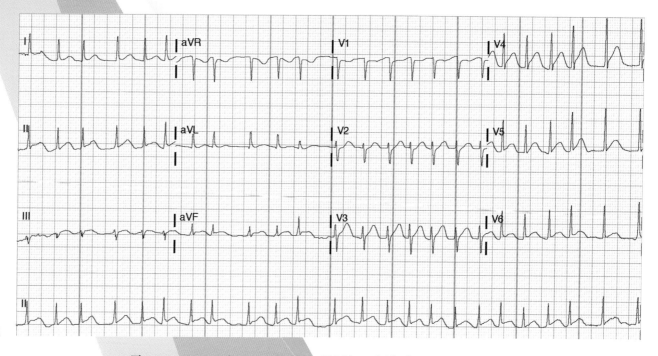

ECG 64.1

There is no prior electrocardiogram (ECG) available for comparison, a repeat ECG was performed (see ECG 64.2).

▸▸ Repeat Electrocardiogram: Would You Activate the Cath Lab?

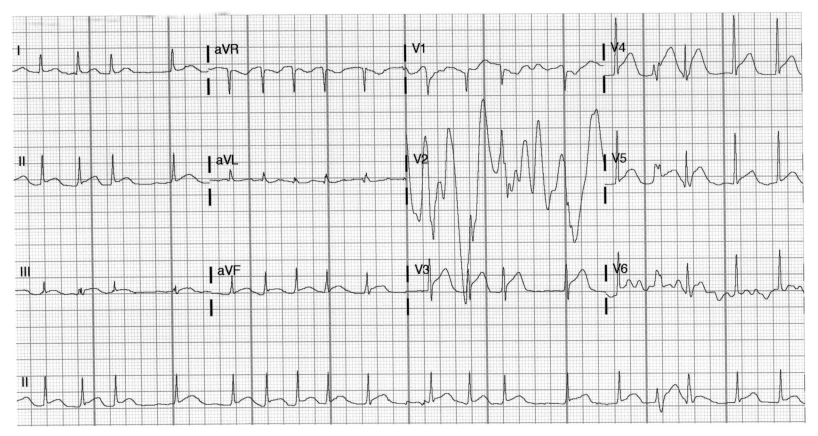

ECG 64.2

EXPLANATION

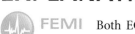 **FEMI** Both ECGs demonstrate atrial fibrillation with rapid ventricular response and anterolateral and inferior ST elevations consistent with acute infarction.

Emergent angiography revealed patent coronary arteries, but marked "sluggish" flow of contrast or significant delayed distal vessel opacification, most prominent in the left anterior descending coronary artery (LAD; anterolateral) and also in the right coronary artery (RCA; inferior) territory—the two coronary distributions that showed ischemia on ECG.

Overall, the ST elevations are not from coronary obstruction but from an acute episode of coronary slow flow phenomenon. This disease entity is believed to originate from microvascular dysfunction, or acute microvascular increases in vascular resistance, leading to reduced filling in the coronary vessels. This disease can cause angina, and has been reported as a cause for ST elevations as in this case due to resulting myocardial ischemia.[1,2]

Treatment with calcium channel blockers may help reduce microvascular resistance and can therefore improve coronary flow in these instances. In fact, as the patient was started on intravenous (IV) diltiazem (a calcium channel blocker) for rate control for atrial fibrillation and the subsequent ECG showed resolution of the ST-segment elevations.

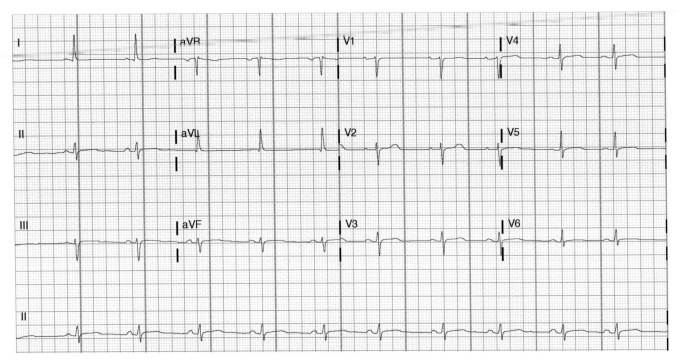

ECG 64.3

See ECG 64.3. Note the spontaneous conversion to sinus rhythm from atrial fibrillation as well as resolution of the ST elevations. It was postulated that the coronary slow flow resulted in significant myocardial ischemic/stress that lead to not only atrial fibrillation but also significant ST contour changes.

References

1. Kapoor A, Goel PK, Gupta S. Slow coronary flow—a cause for angina with ST segment elevation and normal coronary arteries. A case report. *Int J Cardiol.* 1998;67(3):257-261.
2. Sen T. Coronary slow flow phenomenon leads to ST elevation myocardial infarction. *Korean Circ J.* 2013;43(3):196-198.

Case 65

PRESENTATION

A 50-year-old female with history of "a heart attack," stroke, and hypertension presents with acute left-sided chest pain, which radiates to the left arm. She developed this while walking. It is associated with dyspnea and palpitations.

▸▸ **Presenting Electrocardiogram: Would You Activate the Cath Lab?**

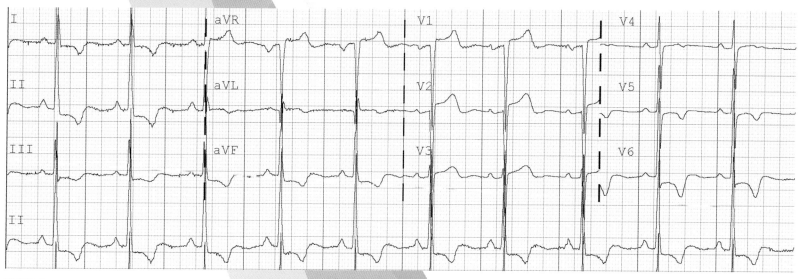

ECG 65.1

A prior electrocardiogram (ECG) is available for comparison (see ECG 65.2).

▶▶ Prior Electrocardiogram for Comparison

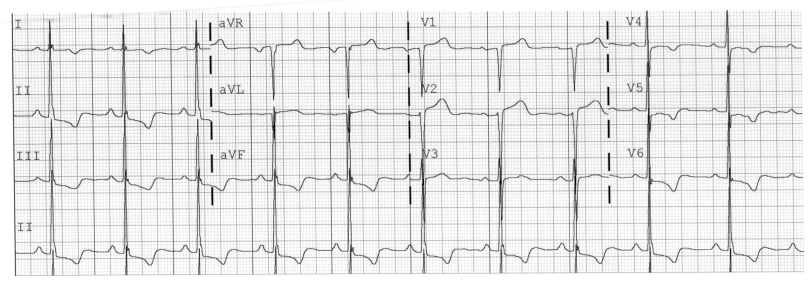

ECG 65.2

EXPLANATION

FEMI The ECG demonstrates sinus rhythm, left atrial enlargement, and left ventricular hypertrophy (LVH) with secondary repolarization with asymmetric T-wave inversions. The degree of ST elevations in leads V_1 and V_2 is concerning for anteroseptal injury.

On emergent catheterization, there was nonobstructive disease. The presenting ECG demonstrates an exaggeration of the ST changes from the baseline ECG (particularly in leads V_1 and V_2). In addition to the new ECG changes, the classic symptoms of acute coronary chest pain, an urgent catheterization was indicated in absence of frank contraindications.

As evident in this case, there are patients who have baseline ST elevations, especially in the context of LVH. Algorithms to adjust for the prominent voltages seen with LVH such as the methodology from the paper by Armstrong et al,[1] the presenting ECG would not suggest ischemia. The amplitude of ST elevation divided by the RS wave in leads V_1, V_2, or V_3 is <25%; acute ischemia is therefore unlikely.[1] However, these proposed methods are not perfect, and sound clinical judgment in the decision-making process in managing acute chest pain remains important.

Review Cases 16, 18, 19, 20, and 45.

Reference

1. Armstrong EJ, Kulkarni AR, Bhave PD, et al. Electrocardiographic criteria for ST-elevation myocardial infarction in patients with left ventricular hypertrophy. *Am J Cardiol.* 2012,110(7):977-983

Case 66

PRESENTATION

A 55-year-old male with hypertension and reported history of a "single kidney" from a congenital condition presents with 1 day of intermittent crushing substernal chest pain, which radiates to the left arm. He had been noncompliant with his medications and his blood pressure was 240/140.

▸▸ **Presenting Electrocardiogram: Would You Activate the Cath Lab?**

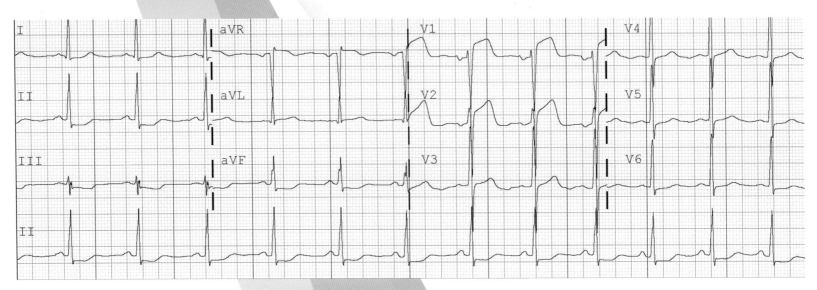

ECG 66.1

A prior electrocardiogram (ECG) is available for comparison (see ECG 66.2).

▶▶ Prior Electrocardiogram for Comparison

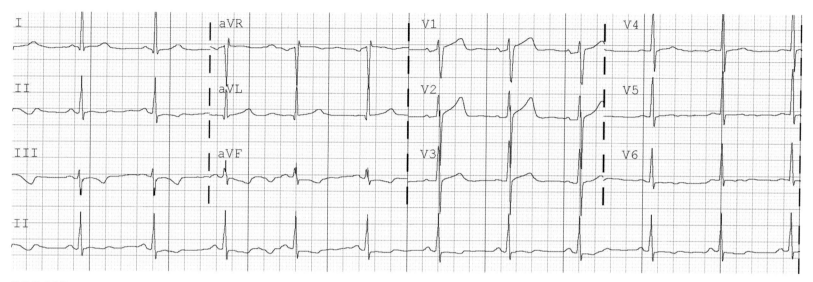

ECG 66.2

EXPLANATION

FEMI The ECG demonstrates left ventricular hypertrophy (LVH) with anteroseptal ST-segment elevations meeting ST-segment elevation myocardial infarction (STEMI) criteria, along with ST elevation in aVR and diffuse ST depression concerning for global ischemia.

The patient was brought for urgent catheterization, but was not found to have an acute culprit lesion. The patient had underlying branch vessel disease including 80% to 90% stenosis in several medium-sized branch vessels including the first and second diagonals, OM_1, OM_2, and the right posterior descending artery (PDA). Because there were no culprit lesions, there was no emergency coronary intervention performed.

The patient remained severely hypertensive and it was postulated that the patient's symptoms and ECG findings were a result of his blood pressure with underlying severe branch vessel coronary artery disease (CAD), leading to "demand ischemia"—supply and demand mismatch. He was transferred to the intensive care unit for management of an acute **hypertensive emergency**. With control of his blood pressure, the patient's symptoms and dramatic ST-T changes were improved (see ECG 66.3).

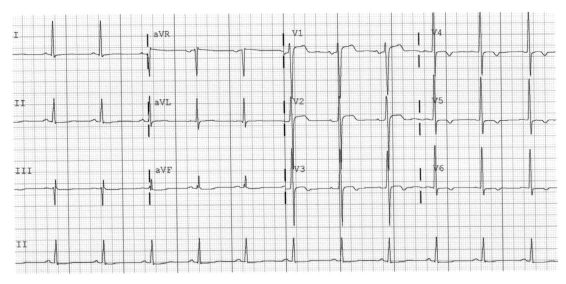

ECG 66.3

Case 67

PRESENTATION

A 52-year-old male without known medical history was brought in by ambulance after a witnessed cardiac arrest. Bystanders were performing cardiopulmonary resuscitation (CPR) prior to Emergency Medical Services arrival. They found the patient to be in ventricular fibrillation (VF), and defibrillated the patient with restoration of sinus rhythm and return of spontaneous circulation.

▸▸ **Presenting Electrocardiogram: Would You Activate the Cath Lab?**

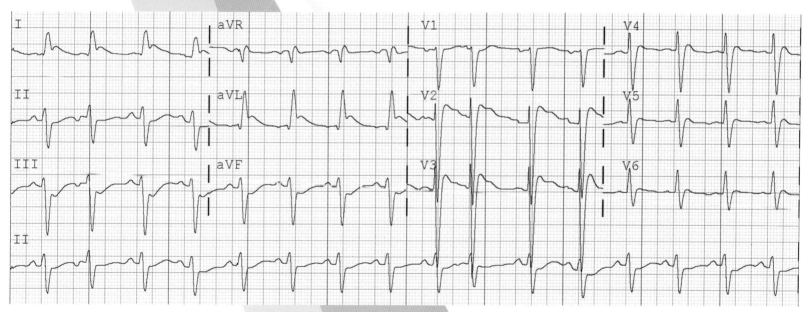

ECG 67.1

There is no prior electrocardiogram (ECG) available for comparison.

EXPLANATION

STEMI   Anterolateral ST-segment elevation myocardial infarction (STEMI) and VF were caused by acute stenosis of the first diagonal artery. In some instances, the branch vessel can subtend enough myocardium to be of significant electrical or hemodynamic consequence.

Selection of appropriate candidate for cardiac catheterization postcardiac arrest is difficult, as the patient may have already suffered prolonged neurologic ischemia, trauma/injury from the fall or from the chest compressions. Post-resuscitation ECGs are often abnormal and may mimic STEMI in morphology due to prolonged hypoxia and subsequent acidosis. However, underlying coronary artery disease (CAD) is present in a most patients presenting with cardiac arrest; the presence of at least 1 significant coronary lesion is an exceedingly common finding in as high as 96% of cases of cardiac arrest due to VF and pulseless VT that presents with an ST elevation on post-resuscitation ECG.[1]

For these reasons, the 2013 American College of Cardiology/American Heart Association (ACC/AHA) STEMI guidelines gave a Class I, Level of Evidence B recommendation for immediate angiography and percutaneous coronary intervention (PCI) for resuscitated out-of-hospital cardiac arrest patients whose initial ECG shows STEMI.[2]

References

1. Dumas F, Cariou A, Manzo-Silberman S, et al. Immediate percutaneous coronary intervention is associated with better survival after out-of-hospital cardiac arrest: insights from the PROCAT (Parisian Region Out of hospital Cardiac ArresT) registry. *Circ Cardiovasc Interv.* 2010;3(3):200-207.
2. Jacobs AK, Kushner FG, Ettinger SM, et al. ACCF/AHA clinical practice guideline methodology summit report: a report of the American College of Cardiology Foundation/American Heart Association Task Force on Practice Guidelines. *J Am Coll Cardiol.* 2013;61(2):213-265.

Case 68

PRESENTATION

A 40-year-old male with type 1 diabetes has been hospitalized in the medical intensive care unit for 2 days for treatment of diabetic ketoacidosis. His glucose and other metabolic parameters have improved and is pending discharge from the intensive care unit.

After returning from the bathroom, the patient reports lightheadedness and diaphoresis. He was quickly brought back to his bed. His blood pressure was 70/50; he had been normotensive throughout his hospital stay.

An electrocardiogram (ECG) was performed and cardiology was urgently consulted.

▸▸ **Presenting Electrocardiogram: Would You Activate the Cath Lab?**

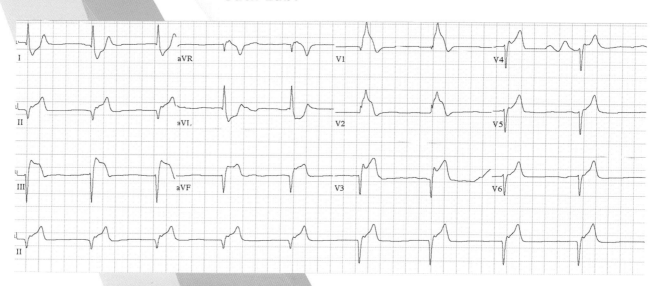

ECG 68.1

A prior ECG is available for comparison (see ECG 68.2).

▶▶ Prior Electrocardiogram for Comparison

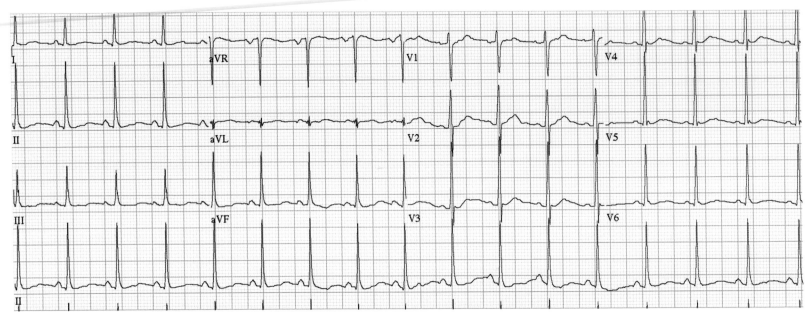

ECG 68.2

EXPLANATION

 FEMI   The ECG demonstrates junctional rhythm with ST elevations in the inferior leads (II, III, aVF), as well as anterior leads (predominantly V_1 to V_4).

As dramatic as these ST changes were, this was a case of massive bilateral pulmonary embolism (noted on autopsy) and not of acute coronary occlusion. After obtaining this ECG, the patient's blood pressure persisted to decline and ultimately the patient developed pulseless electrical activity along with respiratory failure. The patient expired after 40 minutes of unsuccessful resuscitation. Autopsy did not detect significant coronary artery disease.

The classic ECG finding of S1Q3T3 in setting pulmonary embolism was newly present on this ECG. However, the classic signs of right ventricle (RV) strain/compromise including ST depressions and T-wave inversions in leads V_1 to V_4 and leads II, III, aVF were not. However, ST elevations in anteroseptal (and inferior leads) leads were seen, and these lesser common ECG findings in setting of a massive pulmonary embolism have been previously reported.[1,2] A case such as this one is a reminder that marked ST changes do not only arise from coronary artery disease.

Pulmonary embolism can cause ST elevations on ECG via several conceivable mechanisms: (a) acute right ventricular distension leading to compression and decreased blood flow into the right coronary artery, (b) leftward shift of the intraventricular septum in setting of fixed pericardial restraint leading to compression of other coronary arteries including septal perforators, and (c) acute hypoxia.[1]

References

1. Falterman TJ, Martinez JA, Daberkow D, Weiss LD. Pulmonary embolism with ST segment elevation in leads V_1 to V_4: case report and review of the literature regarding electrocardiographic changes in acute pulmonary embolism. *J Emerg Med.* 2001;21(3):255-261.
2. Livaditis IG, Paraschos M, Dimopoulos K. Massive pulmonary embolism with ST elevation in leads V_1-V_3 and successful thrombolysis with tenecteplase. *Heart.* 2004;90(7):e41.

Case 69

PRESENTATION

A 92-year-old female with diabetes, and prior history of stroke and myocardial infarction was found by family unresponsive at home.

Emergency personnel came and found the patient in pulseless electrical arrest (PEA). They began advanced cardiopulmonary resuscitation and the patient achieved return of spontaneous circulation.

On arrival to the emergency department, the following electrocardiogram (ECG) was obtained.

▶▶ **Presenting Electrocardiogram: Would You Activate the Cath Lab?**

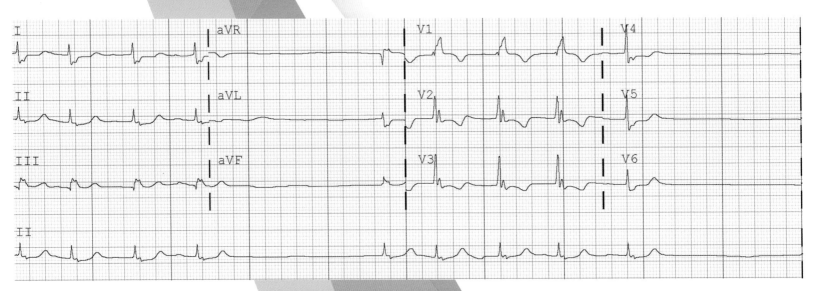

ECG 69.1

There is no prior ECG available for comparison.

EXPLANATION

FEMI   The ECG demonstrates sinus rhythm, first-degree atrioventricular (AV) block, and sinus pauses/arrest with underlying right bundle branch block (RBBB) and left anterior fascicular block (LPFB). There are T-wave inversions in leads V_1 to V_3, which are normal findings in the setting of RBBB.

There is no ischemia suggested. The patient has a primary electrical/conduction issue consistent with sick sinus syndrome with underlying bifascicular block and first-degree AV block. Coronary angiogram is not indicated in this scenario, but instead, urgent initiation of temporary cardiac pacing for symptomatic bradycardia and pauses needs to be considered.

Case 70

PRESENTATION

A 50-year-old male tobacco smoker without previous known cardiac problems presents with acute onset retrosternal chest pain with associated diaphoresis, which started while he was working as a food deliveryman.

▶▶ **Presenting Electrocardiogram: Would You Activate the Cath Lab?**

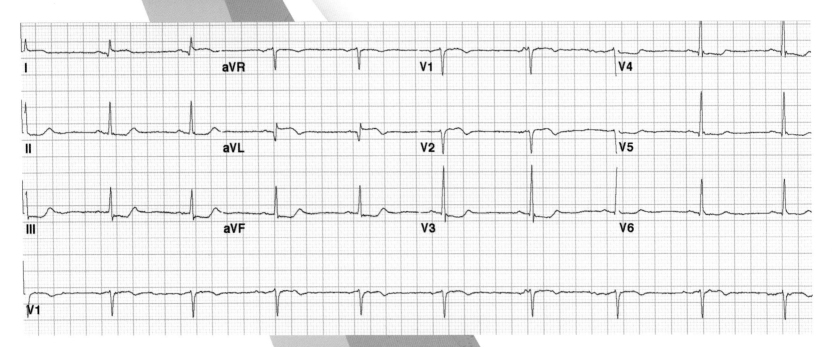

ECG 70.1

There is no prior electrocardiogram (ECG) available for comparison.

EXPLANATION

STEMI   The ECG demonstrates borderline ST elevation in lead I and 1-mm ST elevation in aVL, with reciprocal changes in the inferior leads and anterior/lateral T-wave changes.
This presenting ECG does not meet standard ST-segment elevation myocardial infarction (STEMI)
criteria. It is, however, certainly concerning for an isolated lateral wall infarction. The patient was
indeed found to have a thrombotic occlusion of a fairly large caliber second diagonal artery.

The lateral wall of the left ventricle (LV) is generally supplied by the diagonal branches (of the
left anterior descending coronary artery [LAD]), the obtuse marginal branches (of the left circumflex coronary artery [LCx]), the ramus intermedius (which is an artery that arises from the middle
trifurcation of the left main; this is a normal variant as typically the left main bifurcates into the LAD
and the LCx), or the posterior/lateral branch (of the right coronary artery [RCA]). An isolated lateral
wall infarction is uncommon as typically lateral wall involvement is often a part of a larger anterolateral (LAD) or inferior–posterior–lateral (RCA or LCx) myocardial infarction (MI). Nevertheless,
lateral wall infarction is an indication for emergent angiography.

Typically, infarction of the first diagonal would yield ST elevations in I and aVL and is referred
to a "high lateral MI"; review Case 67. In this case, acute infarction in the second diagonal ("middle
lateral") may have caused the ST elevation in lead I to be less prominent. The anatomic course of the
coronary arteries and ECG lead positioning are factors that influence the ECG signal, and therefore,
may affect the diagnosis.

Case 71

PRESENTATION

A 65-year-old male with hypertension and dyslipidemia presents with escalating midsternal chest pain with radiation to the neck.

▸▸ **Presenting Electrocardiogram: Would You Activate the Cath Lab?**

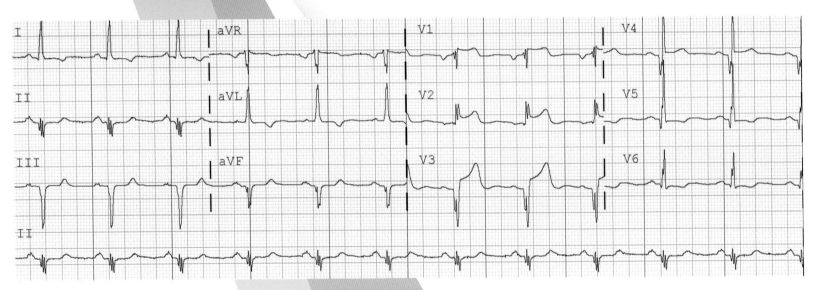

ECG 71.1

There is no prior electrocardiogram (ECG) available for comparison.

EXPLANATION

FEMI   The ECG demonstrates ST elevations with associated Q waves in leads V_1 to V_4 diagnostic of age-indeterminate anteroseptal/anterior infarction. There are also Q waves in the inferior leads suggestive of old inferior infarction.

Despite these ECG changes, there was no acute vessel occlusion. These ST elevations were the result of an underlying left ventricle (LV) aneurysm, which developed as a consequence of a previous proximal left anterior descending coronary artery (LAD) occlusion. Review Case 25. Also, note the fragmented QRS in leads II, V_1, and V_2, which can be suggestive of myocardial scarring.[1]

In subsequent consultation with the patient's outpatient cardiologist, it was discovered that this was a stable ECG pattern. Twenty-four-hour thallium viability study revealed a minimal viable myocardium in the LAD territory, and therefore, an attempt to open the chronically occluded LAD was not performed. To improve overall myocardial perfusion, the patient received angioplasty to a stable 80% mid-left circumflex (LCx) lesion.

One can consider providing patients a copy of their own ECG, especially there is a markedly abnormal baseline.

ECG 71.2

Although having a copy of a baseline ECG can be helpful, occasionally, it still remains diffi-cult to discern if acute ischemia is present simply with an ECG. ECG 71.2 is from a patient with a known large anterior wall aneurysm as a consequence of an LAD infarction, who presented to the hospital after a seizure. Notice the exaggerated anterior ST elevations compared with a prior ECG (see ECG 71.3). An urgent coronary angiogram was performed and demonstrated patent coronary arteries and stents.

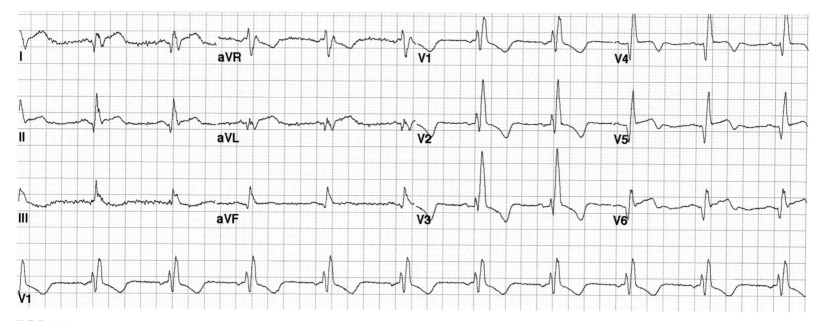

ECG 71.3

Notice that this patient had baseline ST elevations that were less prominent on a prior ECG. Therefore, the ST elevations on presentation were likely an exaggeration during acute stress and possibly some degree of lead placement.

Reference

1. Pietrasik G, Zareba W. QRS fragmentation: diagnostic and prognostic significance. *Cardiol J*. 2012;19(2):114-121.

Case 72

PRESENTATION

The patient in Case 71 returns to the emergency department approximately 6 months later, with recurrence of chest pain symptoms he had presented with previously, but progressive over the past 3 days.

To review, 6 months prior, the patient received a stent placement into the left circumflex. The proximal 100% left anterior descending coronary artery (LAD) occlusion was not treated as the LAD territory did not demonstrate significant viability.

▶▶ **Presenting Electrocardiogram: Would You Activate the Cath Lab?**

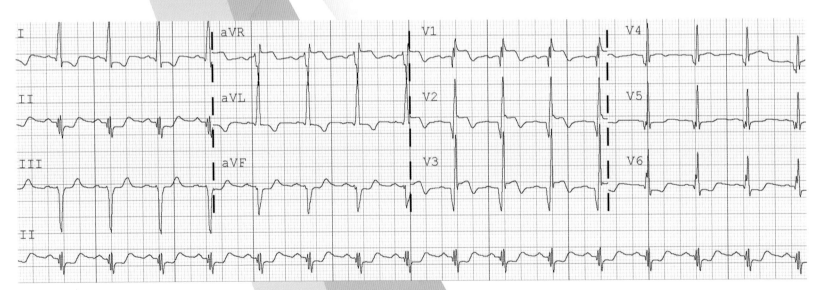

ECG 72.1

A prior electrocardiogram (ECG) is available for comparison (see ECG 72.2).

▶▶ **Prior Electrocardiogram for Comparison**

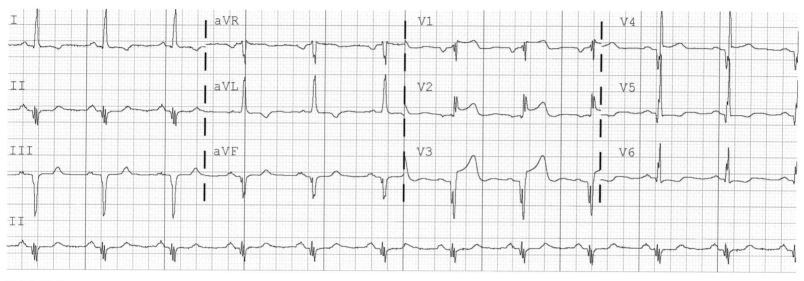

ECG 72.2

EXPLANATION

3TEMI Because the patient's baseline ECG includes ST elevations (from left ventricle [LV] aneurysm), interpretation of additional acute ischemic findings is difficult. This ECG contains not only old ST elevations in V_1 to V_4, but also a new biphasic pattern to the ST-T, tall R-wave anteriorly, as well as new lateral/inferior ST depressions in leads I, II, aVF, and V_6. In addition, there is new ST elevation in aVR.

Coronary angiogram revealed new ostial 90% and distal 60% left main stenosis, and because of this left main lesion, the left circumflex coronary artery (LCx; posterior/lateral) territory was ischemic. The LCx stent was patent, and the proximal LAD remained chronically occluded.

The dramatic progression of disease in the left main within 6 months time is suspicious for catheter-induced coronary artery disease (CAD). Instrumentation with guide catheters, wires, and passage of balloons/stents may damage the intima and instigate accelerated progression of arterial stenosis. In another words, the patient's angioplasty 6 months prior may have traumatized the left main, leading to progressive/accelerated left main CAD, manifesting in an acute coronary syndrome 6 months later. In one study, 9 of 11 autopsy subjects had evidence of left main intimal damage after percutaneous coronary intervention (PCI).[1] **These data remind us that coronary interventions, although often performed and completed successfully, are not completely innocuous.**

Reference

1. Moore S. Endothelial injury and atherosclerosis. *Exp Mol Pathol.* 1979;31(1):182-190.

Case 73

PRESENTATION

A 73-year-old male with hypertension, dyslipidemia, and acid reflux presents with several weeks of intermittent left-sided chest pain. The pain was sharp in quality, non-radiating, and not related to any activity.

On further questioning, he reports undergoing cardiac catheterizations 4 times in the past several years. He reports, "they found nothing" every time. The patient seems to receive care intermittently at many different hospitals.

▸▸ **Presenting Electrocardiogram: Would You Activate the Cath Lab?**

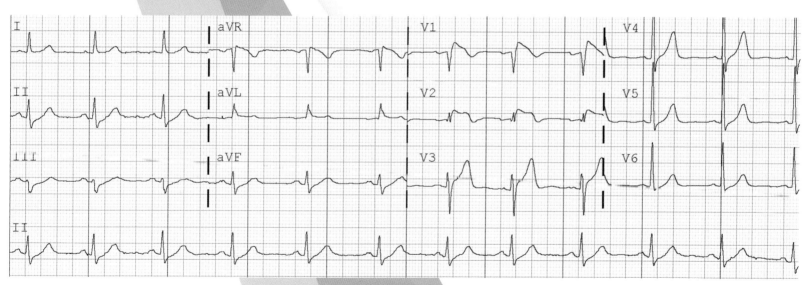

ECG 73.1

A prior electrocardiogram (ECG) is available for comparison (see ECG 73.2).

▶▶ Prior Electrocardiogram for Comparison

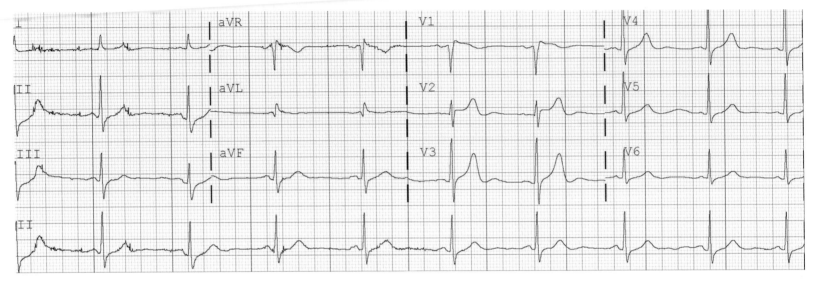

ECG 73.2

EXPLANATION

FEMI   The ECG demonstrates Q waves, fractionated QRS, and ST elevations in V_1 and V_2, concerning for age-indeterminate anteroseptal infarction, with ST depressions in the inferior leads concerning inferior involvement.

Cardiology was urgently consulted. After review of the medical record, it became clear that the patient had atypical chest pain symptoms and had an asymptomatic Brugada "Type II" pattern on ECG. The patient's fifth lifetime cardiac catheterization was prevented.

The Brugada pattern on ECG is in large a result of abnormal ion channel function, and not indicative of myocardial ischemia. The presence of a Brugada pattern on ECG without associated clinical features (ie, Brugada syndrome) such as ventricular arrhythmias, family history of sudden cardiac death, or unexplained syncope may be of questionable significance. The Brugada pattern may at times be more pronounced than at other times—with potential inciting factors such as fever, electrolyte imbalance, lead placement, or true ischemia. Note how the ST elevation in lead V_2 was not present on the prior ECG. *One may consider providing the patient with a copy of his or her own "abnormal ECG" as a reference for future physician encounters* (Figure 73.1 depicts the three recognized Brugada patterns).

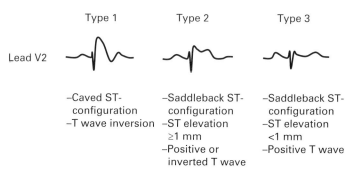

Figure 73.1

Figure adapted from Antzelevitch et al.[1]

ST-segment contour changes of the Brugada pattern mimic that of ST elevations due to myocardial ischemia; recognize the similarities and differences (see ECGs 73.3 and 73.4).

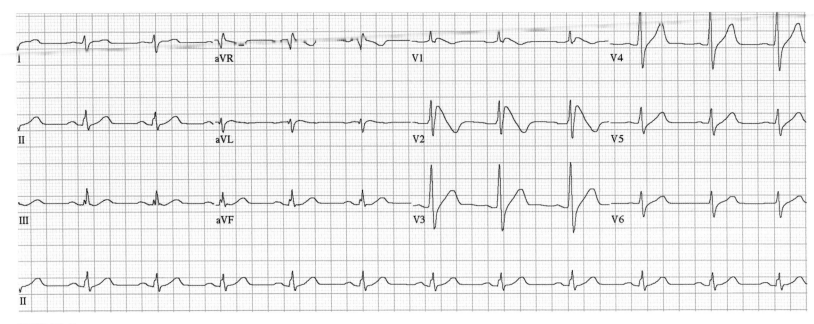

ECG 73.3

ECG 73.3 is an example of Type I Brugada pattern is discovered in a 34-year-old male with fever and sepsis. At baseline, the patient has a normal ECG without the ST-contour changes in leads V_1 and V_2. Conditions that could potentially unmask ECG findings of Brugada syndrome include fever, hyper/hypokalemia, medications with sodium channel blocking properties, and alcohol/cocaine abuse.[1]

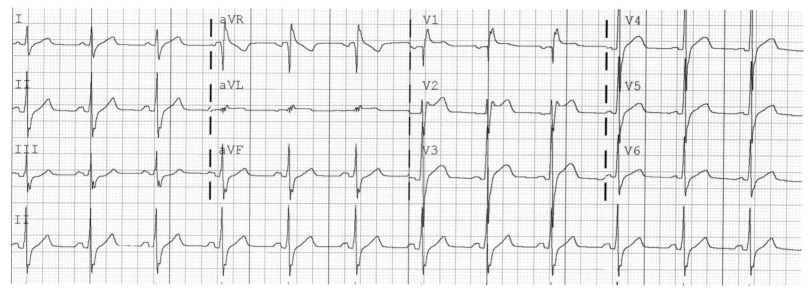

ECG 73.4

ECG 73.4 is an example from another case where there was an initial concern for coronary ischemia. On closer inspection, the patient's ECG is consistent with "Type 2" Brugada pattern.

Reference

1. Antzelevitch C, Brugada P, Borggrefe M, et al. Brugada syndrome: report of the second consensus conference: endorsed by the Heart Rhythm Society and the European Heart Rhythm Association. *Circulation.* 2005;111(5):659-670.

Case 74

PRESENTATION

A 48-year-old male without known cardiac history presents with palpitations. On the morning of presentation, he reports having had some chest pressure along with the sensation of a "rapid heart rate."

▸▸ **Presenting Electrocardiogram: Would You Activate the Cath Lab?**

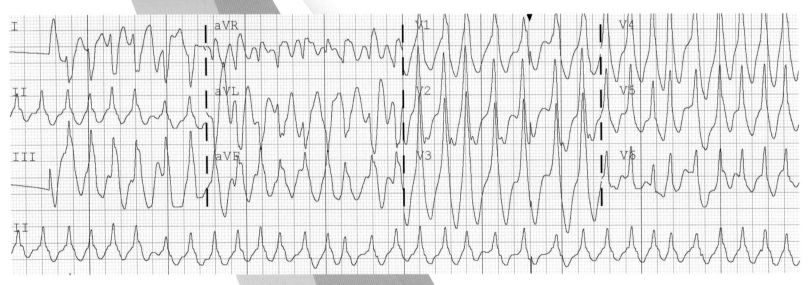

ECG 74.1

There is no prior electrocardiogram (ECG) available for comparison.

EXPLANATION

FEMI   This ECG is classic for preexcitation atrial fibrillation with the rapid, irregular heart, and variable QRS segment duration. This is a result of ventricular fusion beats triggered by irregular (ie, atrial fibrillation) electrical impulses traveling randomly and competitively down both the native atrioventricular (AV) node and through an accessory pathway.

The presenting rhythm was a supraventricular tachycardia and not ventricular tachycardia/fibrillation. The patient had rapid atrial fibrillation with underlying preexcitation, Wolff–Parkinson–White syndrome.

In these instances, administration of adenosine (or other AV nodal blocking agents) can be fatal—blocking the AV node would favor the electrical impulse down the accessory pathway, which can lead to extremely fast heart rates with ultimate degeneration into ventricular fibrillation. The patient was electrically cardioverted to sinus rhythm and a repeat ECG was performed.

ECG was obtained after electro-cardioversion to sinus rhythm (see ECG 74.2).

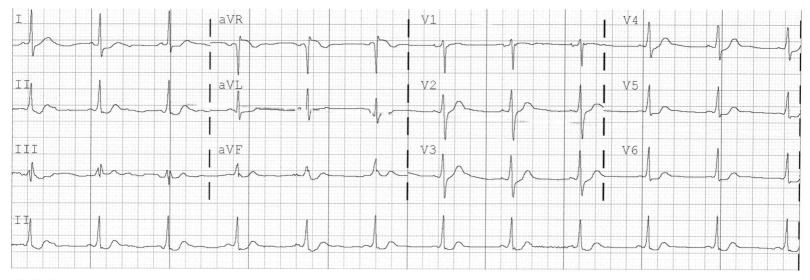

ECG 74.2

?

Should the patient undergo an emergent cardiac catheterization?
1. No. The ECG after electrocardioversion demonstrates sinus rhythm and diffuse ST depression with ST elevation in lead aVR; however, in this clinical context, these transient ischemic changes are caused by the rapid ventricular rates (close to 200 beats per minute) that occurred for such sustained period. The patient's arrhythmia was not triggered by coronary ischemia.
2. Note the "delta wave" and short PR interval, which is ECG evidence of manifested preexcitation. The patient subsequently underwent ablation of a left lateral accessory pathway. ECG evidence of preexcitation is eliminated on the post-ablation ECG; see ECG 74.3.

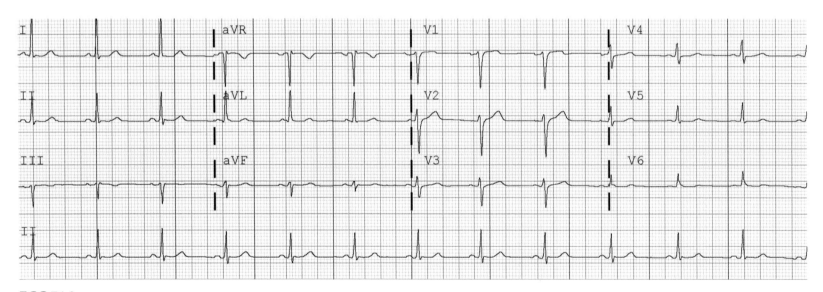

ECG 74.3

ECG post-ablation of left lateral accessory pathway. Note the absence of the delta waves and short PR interval.

Case 75

PRESENTATION

A 66-year-old male with lifelong tobacco abuse, without known coronary artery disease (CAD) presents for a parotidectomy for localized malignancy. After an uncomplicated surgery and while recovering from anesthesia, the patient reported acute chest pain and alerted the nurses. The chest pressure was sustained for 20 to 30 minutes, with numbness sensation that radiated to the bilateral arms. An electrocardiogram (ECG) was performed.

▸▸ **Presenting Electrocardiogram: Would You Activate the Cath Lab?**

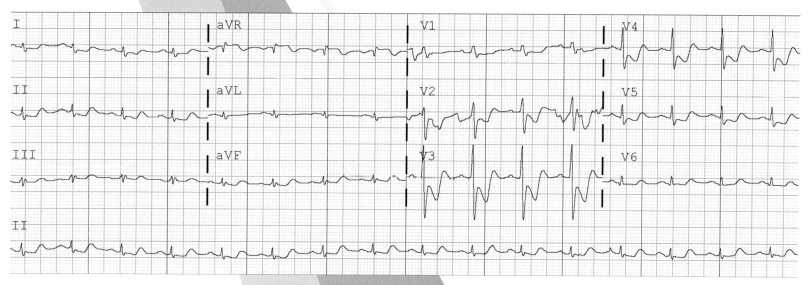

ECG 75.1

A prior ECG is available for comparison (see ECG 75.2).

▶▶ Prior Electrocardiogram for Comparison

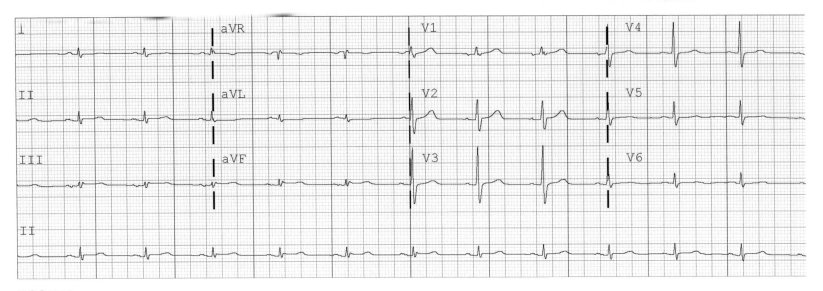

ECG 75.2

If you did not activate the catheterization laboratory, when would you postpone a cardiac catheterization until?

EXPLANATION

STEMI   Although the presenting ECG does not meet ECG criteria for ST-segment elevation myocardial infarction (STEMI), the findings of "high-risk" global dramatic ST-T changes with ST elevation in lead aVR should not be ignored. **This case is not a STEMI by conventional definitions, but its urgency is similar and therefore will be categorized as such.**

The ECG performed on the next day was essentially unremarkable (see ECG 75.3), which was perhaps falsely reassuring as no further action was pursued. Four days post-operation, the patient developed a cardiac arrest, resuscitated, and was emergently sent for cardiac catheterization. Severe diffuse triple vessel disease with an unstable proximal left anterior descending coronary artery (LAD) stenosis was diagnosed; coronary bypass surgery was performed.

The evaluation of chest pain in the immediate postsurgical patient is difficult, as the patient will inevitably be clouded by postoperative pain and the lingering effects of sedatives/anesthetics. Often times, much is relied on the patient's hemodynamics, vital signs, and adjunctive diagnostic tests (ie, the ECG). Adjunctive postoperative screening tests with ECG (especially if chest pain symptoms occur postsurgically) can be very helpful in ruling out significant postoperative cardiovascular morbidity, which can be triggered by the stress of surgery.

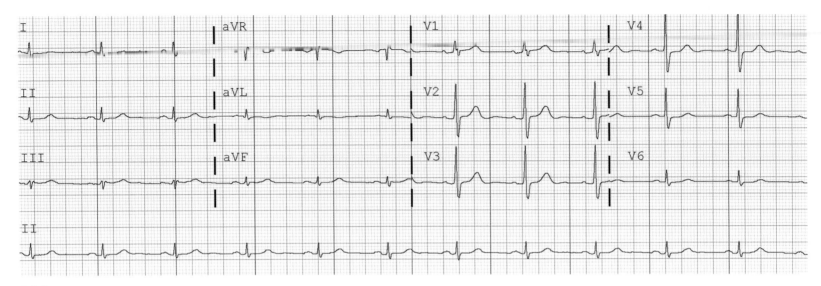

ECG 75.3

ECG 75.3 shows the ECG that was performed 1 day post-operation. The postoperative "Wellens'-like" T wave resolved (as did the chest pain), however, the initial ECG changes should not be ignored—especially if there are no contraindications for cardiac catheterization. In the original Wellens' study, biphasic/deeply inverted anterior T waves were highly associated with a critical proximal LAD lesion.[1] Review Cases 8 and 22.

Reference

1. de Zwaan C, Bär FW, Wellens HJ. Characteristic electrocardiographic pattern indicating a critical stenosis high in left anterior descending coronary artery in patients admitted because of impending myocardial infarction. *Am Heart J.* 1982;103(4, pt 2):730-736.

Case 76

PRESENTATION

A 47-year-old male without known cardiac history presented with a 2-minute episode of crushing chest pain. This occurred as the patient was being arrested by police for shoplifting. As the pain diminished, there was a lingering component of shortness of breath and persistent low-grade substernal discomfort. The patient was therefore transported to a local hospital.

▸▸ **Presenting Electrocardiogram: Would You Activate the Cath Lab?**

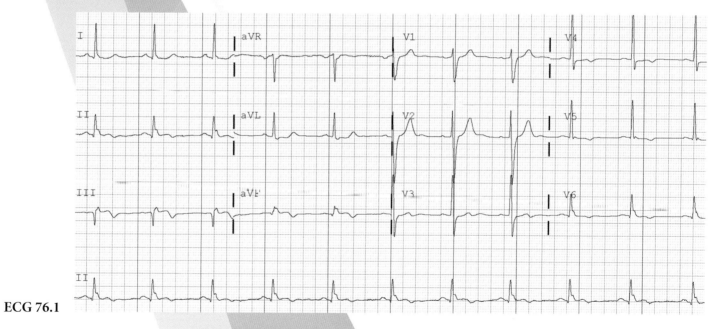

ECG 76.1

There is no prior electrocardiogram (ECG) available for comparison, a repeat ECG was performed (see ECG 76.2).

▶▶ Repeat Electrocardiogram: Would You Activate the Cath Lab?

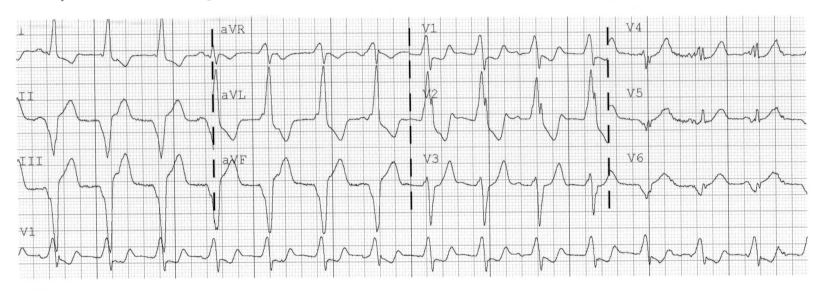

ECG 76.2

EXPLANATION

STEMI The presenting ECG demonstrates <1-mm ST elevations in leads II, III, and aVF but with ischemic appearing ST changes/contours. The second ECG demonstrates accelerated idioventricular rhythm (AIVR). In setting of suspected ischemia, this rhythm generally denotes myocardial injury via coronary occlusion. The presence of this rhythm does not necessarily imply complete vessel patency or resolution of an unstable plaque, and therefore a potential indication for urgent cardiac catheterization. **Although none of the ECGs met ST-segment elevation myocardial infarction (STEMI) criteria, this case will be categorized as STEMI to highlight the need for recognition of coronary occlusion in setting of an ischemic ECG and subsequent development of AIVR.** The patient indeed had an unstable appearing distal right coronary artery (RCA) stenosis on catheterization.

Historically, AIVR is regarded as a "reperfusion rhythm" in patients treated with fibrinolytics.[1] In the era of prompt primary percutaneous coronary intervention (PCI), this most common post-myocardial infarction (MI) rhythm may actually suggest extensive myocardial damaged and delayed microvascular reperfusion.[2] Either way, AIVR (a form of "slow monomorphic ventricular tachycardia") classically occurs in setting of acute myocardial infarction when there is concomitant increased vagal tone with decreased sympathetic tone. Hence, AIVR is more commonly seen with inferior–posterior MIs, which can elicit the Bezold–Jarisch reflex (increased vagal tone secondary to ischemia) and bradycardia.

References

1. Krumholz HM, Goldberger AL. Reperfusion arrhythmias after thrombolysis. Electrophysiologic tempest, or much ado about nothing. *Chest.* 1991;99(4 Suppl):135S-140S.
2. Terkelsen CJ, Sørensen JT, Kaltoft AK, et al. Prevalence and significance of accelerated idioventricular rhythm in patients with ST-elevation myocardial infarction treated with primary percutaneous coronary intervention. *Am J Cardiol.* 2009;104(12):1641-1646.

Case 77

PRESENTATION

A 65-year-old female with hypertension, dyslipidemia, and diastolic heart failure is brought to the emergency department for chest pain. The initial electrocardiogram (ECG) showed narrow complex regular tachycardia with heart rates in the 160s. She was noted to be hypotensive to 90/50.

The emergency department was concerned about the ST elevation in lead aVR and the ischemic ST-T contours on multiple leads.

▶▶ **Presenting Electrocardiogram: Would You Activate the Cath Lab?**

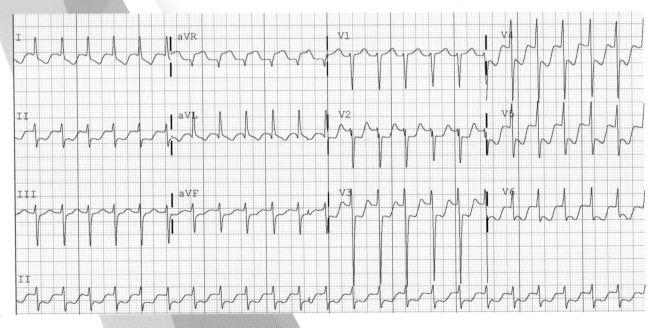

ECG 77.1

There is no prior ECG available for comparison.

EXPLANATION

FEMI   The ECG demonstrates a supraventricular tachycardia (SVT) with diffuse ST-T ischemic depressions and ST elevation in lead aVR. Although the presenting ECG was not an ST-segment elevation myocardial infarction (STEMI), it was indeed a "high-risk" ECG indicative of global myocardial ischemia. But, this was not a case of acute coronary syndrome.

After review of her medical record, it was noted the patient had underlying critical aortic stenosis (with an estimated valve area 0.6 cm^2). Therefore, while there was global sub-endomyocardial ischemia on the ECG, this is consistent with the consequences of her aortic stenosis in the setting of an SVT. Termination of the SVT was the next step, not coronary angiography. Indeed, with restoration of normal sinus rhythm, the blood pressure improved as well as the ST-T changes. Review Case 5.

Important to note is that ST-segment changes in setting of SVT do not always indicate underlying obstructive coronary artery disease (CAD); patients proven to not to have obstructive CAD may still demonstrate ST changes with SVT. The ST-segment changes are likely a result of sustained oxygen supply and demand mismatch as a consequence of tachycardia.

Reference

1. Güleç S, Ertas F, Karaoouz R, Güldal M, Alpman A, Oral D. Value of ST-segment depression during paroxysmal supraventricular tachycardia in the diagnosis of coronary artery disease. *Am J Cardiol.* 1999;83(3):458-460, A10.

Case 78

PRESENTATION

A 69-year-old female with diabetes and hypertension presents from home with 2 hours of increasing retrosternal chest discomfort and progressive weakness. En route to the hospital, emergency medical services noted abnormal electrocardiogram (ECG) concerning for acute infarction.

On arrival to the emergency department, she developed progressive hypotension and required intubation for impending respiratory failure. As her airway was secured, her blood tests returned and the serum potassium was elevated at 6.4 mmol/L (normal range is 3.5 to 5.0 mmol/L).

▶▶ **Presenting Electrocardiogram: Would You Activate the Cath Lab?**

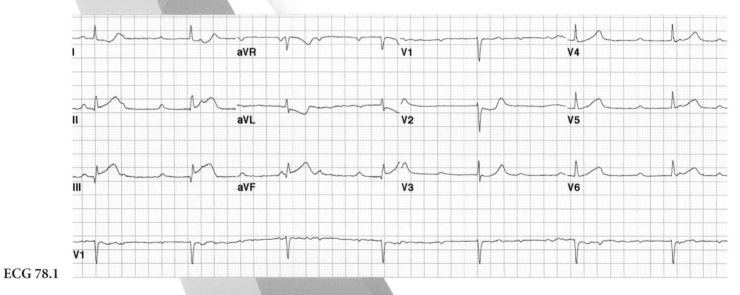

ECG 78.1

There is no prior ECG available for comparison.

EXPLANATION

STEMI   The presenting ECG demonstrates sinus rhythm with complete heart block and inferior ST elevations, consistent inferior myocardial infarction (MI) with posterior extension.

Despite the elevated serum potassium, there were no clear ECG signs of hyperkalemia. Note that hyperkalemia may give rise to peak T waves with horizontal ST segment, where the presenting ECG demonstrates broaden T waves with convex ST elevations. Review Cases 44 and 63. The patient's hyperkalemia is likely a result of the hypotension and acute right ventricular (RV) infarction.

From a cardiac catheterization perspective, hyperkalemia may pose increased risk of provoking malignant arrhythmias and is regarded as a relative contraindication.[1] Nevertheless, emergent cardiac catheterization was deemed necessary as prompt revascularization and obtaining appropriate hemo-dynamic information would afford the best opportunity to stabilize the patient. Electrolytes were monitored with close attention post-procedure. Her cardiac status improved with revascularization and medical management of RV infarction including volume repletion and a brief period of inotrope support.

Reference

1.   Kern MJ. *The Cardiac Catheterization Handbook.* 5th ed. Philadelphia, PA: Elsevier Saunders; 2011:4.

Case 79

PRESENTATION

A 34-year-old male with traumatic brain injury with previous brain surgery and ongoing polysubstance abuse presents from home to the emergency department after he was found unresponsive. There were concerns for seizure-like activity while in the emergency department, and the patient was intubated for airway instability.

He was found to be febrile, with evidence of mild rhabdomyolysis but with normal serum creatinine. An electrocardiogram (ECG) was performed. A troponin was also sent, which returned elevated at 17 ng/mL (normal range is <0.01 ng/mL).

▸▸ **Presenting Electrocardiogram: Would You Activate the Cath Lab?**

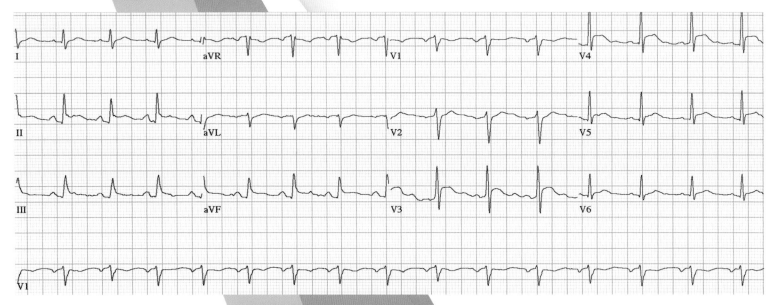

ECG 79.1

There is no prior ECG available for comparison, a repeat ECG was performed (see ECG 79.2).

▶▶ Repeat Electrocardiogram: Would You Activate the Cath Lab?

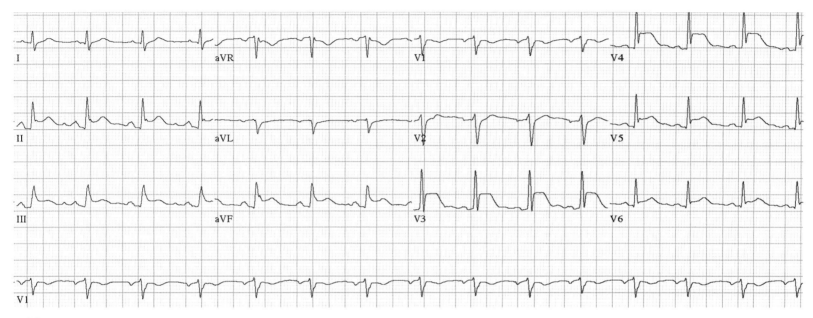

ECG 79.2

EXPLANATION

FFMI There are indeed ST elevations in the anterior and inferior leads consistent with anterior/inferior infarction, which would be consistent with the serum troponin levels. However, cardiac catheterization revealed normal coronaries with normal left ventricular (LV) function.

With these striking ECG findings, it is difficult to ignore the potential for underlying severe acute coronary artery disease. Despite having multiple active and chronic medical issues, there were no frank contraindications for angiography. **Sometimes, it is simply impossible to differentiate an acute coronary syndrome from its mimics.**

The final diagnosis was myopericarditis, as there also appears to have diffuse ST changes with subtle PR depressions (which may be a result of atrial subepicardial injury).

Case 80

PRESENTATION

A 47-year-old male with asthma presents with sudden onset chest pain with occasional pain radiating to the back. A computed tomography (CT) of the chest was ordered to rule out an aortic dissection.

▸▸ **Presenting Electrocardiogram: Would You Activate the Cath Lab?**

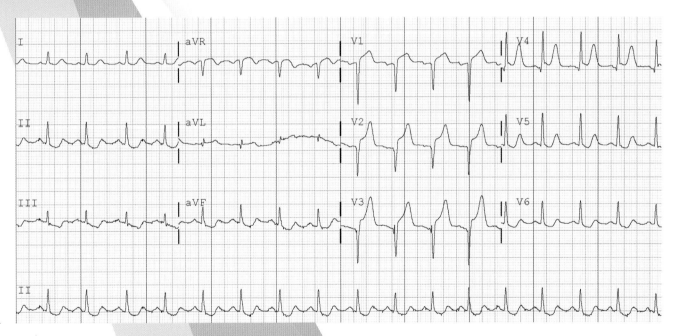

ECG 80.1

There is no prior electrocardiogram (ECG) available for comparison, a repeat ECG was performed (see ECG 80.2).

▶▶ Repeat Electrocardiogram: Would You Activate the Cath Lab?

The patient reports improved symptoms. CT chest was negative for an aortic dissection.

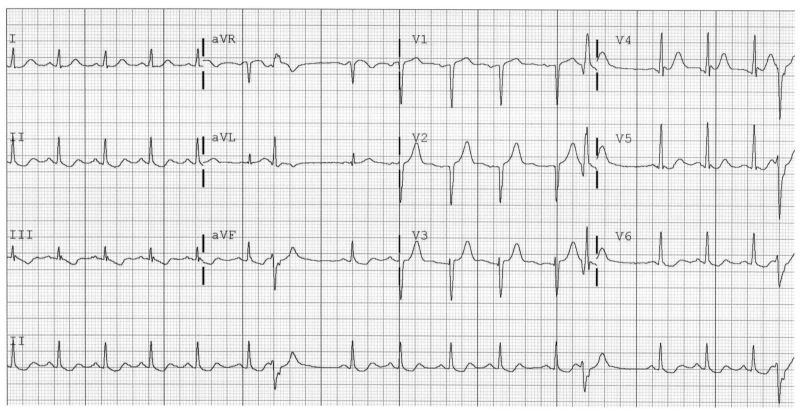

ECG 80.2

EXPLANATION

STEMI The initial ECG showed anterior ST elevations with the peaked T waves suggestive of infarction; however, on the repeat ECG within 10 minutes, these findings were less prominent. These "reassuring" ECG changes and the concerning back pain described by the patient led to the decision to delay cardiac catheterization and proceed with CT scan first to rule out aortic dissection. As the CT scan was noted to be negative for aortic dissection, the troponin results had returned as elevated. The patient was then sent for catheterization, which revealed a culprit diffuse proximal left anterior descending coronary artery (LAD) 95% stenosis.

This case illustrates caution in activating emergent cardiac catheterization where myocardial ischemia was suspected, along with suspected concomitant aortic disease. Review Cases 47 and 48.

The improvement of the anterior ECG changes between the initial and second ECGs likely represents *spontaneous coronary reperfusion* of a culprit artery. This phenomenon is believed to occur in up to 15% of ST-segment elevation myocardial infarctions (STEMIs), and may be assisted by medical therapy including aspirin. Spontaneous reperfusion can be classified via ECG (ie, ≥70% ST-segment resolution) or via angiogram (ie, spontaneous reestablishment of thrombolysis in myocardial infarction (TIMI) 3 flow, which is normal coronary flow via angiographic assessment)—this patient had ≥70% ST-segment resolution on this patient's second ECG.[1]

Despite objective evidence of spontaneous reperfusion, proceeding with catheterization is of importance as there may still be an obstructive unstable stenosis requiring therapy, as in this case.

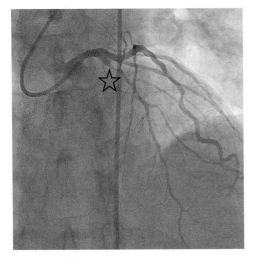

Figure 80.1

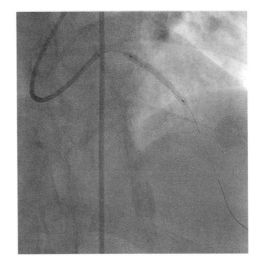

Figure 80.2

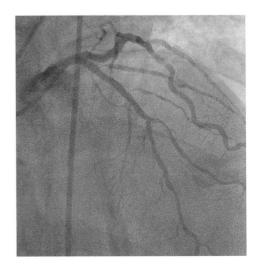

Figure 80.3

Spontaneous regression of ST elevation seen on the repeat serial ECG likely represents spontaneous coronary reperfusion—whether as a result of naturally present anticoagulants or from medical therapy. Despite spontaneous reperfusion, there was still high-grade stenosis with reduced coronary flow through the proximal LAD lesion (*blue star*), which was treated with angioplasty and stenting.

Reference

1. Bainey KR, Fu Y, Wagner GS, et al.; ASSENT 4 PCI Investigators. Spontaneous reperfusion in ST-elevation myocardial infarction: comparison of angiographic and electrocardiographic assessments. *Am Heart J.* 2008;156(2):248-255.

Case 81

PRESENTATION

A 49-year-old male with hypertension, family history of premature coronary artery disease, and heavy lifelong tobacco use presents after an episode of chest pain after lifting heavy items at a parade. It was acute onset, left sided, "crushing" in nature, and not associated with any nausea or vomiting.

▸▸ **Presenting Electrocardiogram: Would You Activate the Cath Lab?**

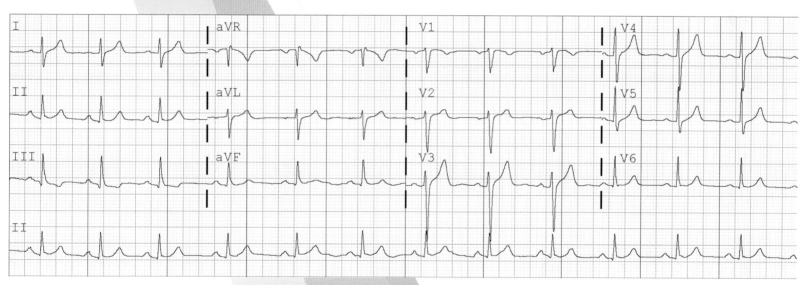

ECG 81.1

There is no prior electrocardiogram (ECG) available for comparison, a repeat ECG was performed (see ECG 81.2).

▶▶ Repeat Electrocardiogram: Would You Activate the Cath Lab?

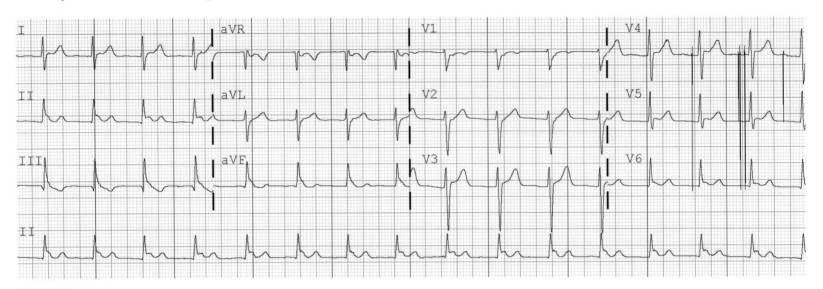

ECG 81.2

EXPLANATION

FEMI   At first glance, one may notice a change in the ST-segment morphology in the inferior leads on the repeat ECG. However, on closer inspection, the second ECG demonstrates an accelerated junctional rhythm with retrograde P waves superimposed on the ST segment.

An alert for emergent cardiac catheterization was signaled when the second ECG was noted, but was cancelled on recognizing this arrhythmia. The patient ultimately had a negative stress test and was discharged from the emergency department.

This case reinforces the importance of exercising a systematic approach at interpreting ECGs (ie, rate, rhythm, morphology), which may, in this example, help provide an explanation for ST-T abnormalities. Another similar scenario can be seen with atrial flutter or atrial fibrillation where the "coarse fibrillatory" waves are superimposed onto the ST segments, giving the illusion of ischemic ST changes.

Case 82

PRESENTATION

A 56-year-old male with polysubstance abuse and metastatic lung adenocarcinoma that was diagnosed 2 weeks ago, reportedly metastatic to the bone, presents with acutely worsening of chest pain along with diffuse body ache. The chest pain was not pleuritic, reproducible, or positional. On examination, he was in obvious distress. The patient has not begun oncologic treatment.

▸▸ **Presenting Electrocardiogram: Would You Activate the Cath Lab?**

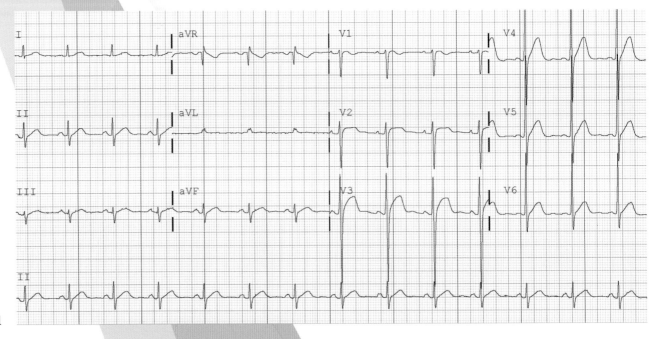

ECG 82.1

A prior electrocardiogram (ECG) is available for comparison (see ECG 82.2).

▶▶ Prior Electrocardiogram for Comparison

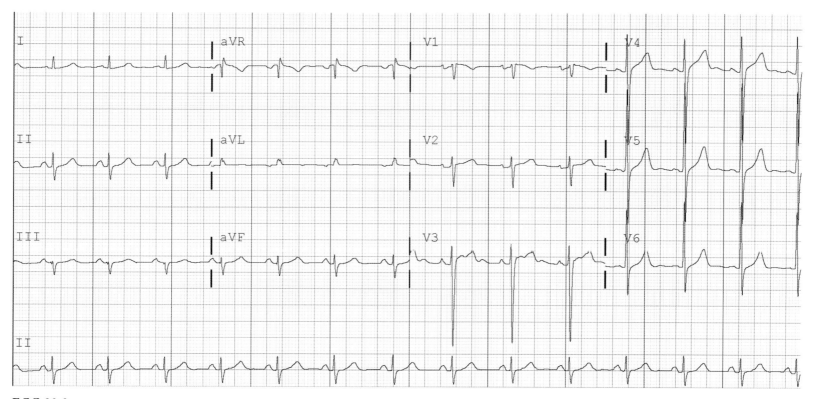

ECG 82.2

EXPLANATION

 FEMI The presenting ECG demonstrates new convex anterior ST-segment contour changes in leads V_2 and V_3, which is indeed concerning for ischemia.

Catheterization, however, revealed normal coronaries.

The patient had hypercalcemia of malignancy, with serum calcium level of 19.8 mg/dL (*normal range is 8.5 to 10.3 mg/dL*). Slight QT-segment shortening from baseline can be noted on the ECG.

Metabolic derangements (eg, hypercalcemia and hyperkalemia) can yield ST-segment changes on ECG. The patient had multiple lytic lesions that are seen throughout the ribs, sternum, and left scapula on chest x-ray performed in the emergency department—his pain could have been associated with these skeletal lesions. Intravenous hydration and Pamidronate were administered, both of which reduced the serum calcium level, and the ECG findings resolved.

This case illustrates how "convex" ST-segment changes, often used to describe the ST-segment changes of myocardial infarction, can be a fake ST-segment elevation myocardial infarction (FEMI).

Case 83

PRESENTATION

A 71-year-old male with advanced systolic heart failure on home milrinone therapy, left ventricular ejection fraction of 15%, coronary artery disease, and atrial fibrillation presents with respiratory distress. There was some report of chest discomfort, but by the time emergency medical services arrived to the patient's home, he became unresponsive, hypoxic (oxygen saturations 70%), and hypotensive.

An electrocardiogram (ECG) was obtained en route to the hospital and there is concern for an acute myocardial infarction (MI).

▶▶ **Presenting Electrocardiogram: Would You Activate the Cath Lab?**

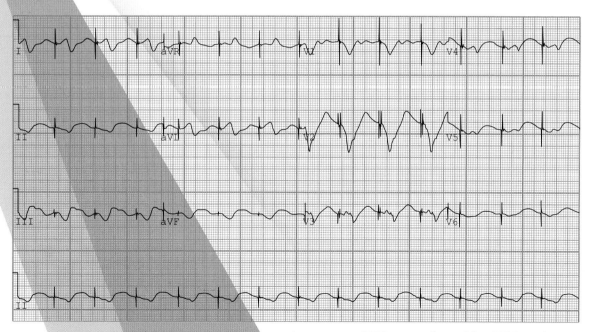

ECG 83.1

There is no prior ECG available for comparison, a repeat ECG was performed (see ECG 83.2).

▶▶ Repeat Electrocardiogram: Would You Activate the Cath Lab?

Vent rate	97 bpm	Demand pacemaker with interpretation is based on intrinsic rhythm
PR interval	* ms	Atrial fibrillation with premature aberrantly conducted complexes
QRS duration	88 ms	Indetermante axis
QT/QTc	220/279 ms	Pulmonary disease pattern
P-R-T axis	* 0 –85	ST elevation consider lateral injury or acute infarct
		** ** ACUTE MI ** **
		Abnormal ECG

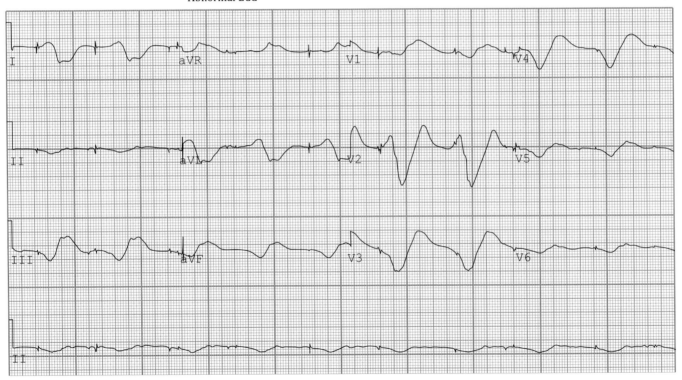

ECG 83.2

EXPLANATION

 FEMI The ECG demonstrates biventricular pacing pattern with a markedly widened QRS with a prolonged QT interval.

While the software had interpreted the ECG as being consistent with an acute infarction pattern, the patient actually had hyperkalemia resulting in bizarrely widened QRS and nearly sinusoidal waves on the repeat ECG. Serum potassium was 7.1 mmol/L (*normal range is 3.5 to 5.0 mmol/L*). The patient had acute kidney injury in setting of worsening of systolic heart failure despite milrinone therapy, leading to the rise in serum potassium. The diagnosis of ST-segment elevation myocardial infarction (STEMI) in a right ventricle (RV)-paced or biventricular-paced rhythm can be very difficult; however, the bizarre appearing and extremely wide QRS duration should be suspicious for underlying metabolic derangements rather than acute MI. This case illustrates the importance of confirming automated ECG interpretations. Review Cases 44, 63, and 78.

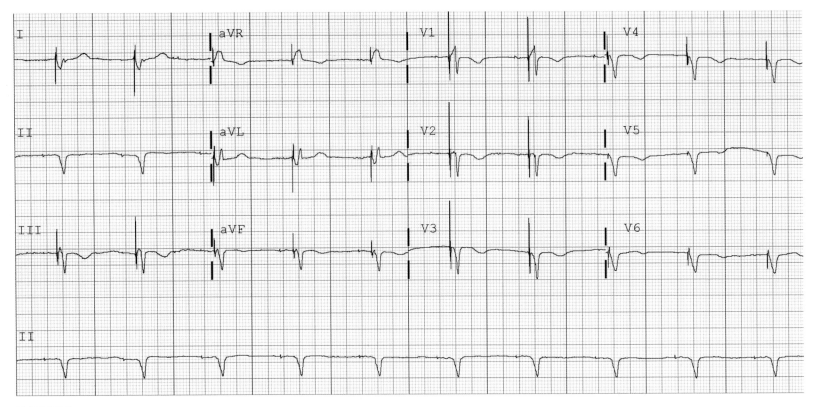

ECG 83.3

ECG 83.3 shows a patient with normal biventricular pacing.

Case 84

PRESENTATION

A 76-year-old female with hypertension and dyslipidemia presents with acute onset chest pain while work. The pain is described as pressure-like and radiating of the pain to the left arm.

▶▶ **Presenting Electrocardiogram: Would You Activate the Cath Lab?**

If you answer "yes" to activate the Catheterization laboratory, which vessel (left main [LM], left anterior descending coronary artery [LAD], left circumflex coronary artery [LCx], or right coronary artery [RCA]) would you anticipate as the culprit vessel?

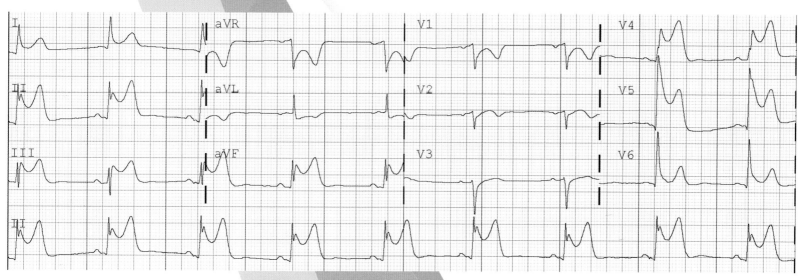

ECG 84.1

There is no prior electrocardiogram (ECG) available for comparison.

EXPLANATION

STEMI   The ECG demonstrates ST elevations in the anterior and inferior leads.
The culprit vessel was the mid-LAD. *But, why were there ST elevations in the inferior leads?*

From a coronary anatomy standpoint, the patient's LAD was a "wraparound" LAD, meaning that the LAD wraps around the left ventricle (LV) apex and continues in its course to supply blood to the inferior wall of the LV. Therefore, with LAD occlusion, not only will it cause the expected anterior ischemia, but also inferior wall ischemia. Review Case 37.

Conversely, there are cases where the RCA is a large dominant vessel that it can wraparound into the antero/apical and lateral walls of the heart (and accounting for the antero/lateral ST elevations in setting of an RCA ST-segment elevation myocardial infarction [STEMI]).

This is a case in point of how ECGs do not always accurately localize the culprit vessel. But to the ECG's defense, ECGs are merely diagnostic tests.

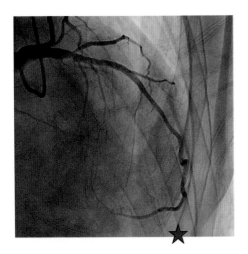

Figure 84.1

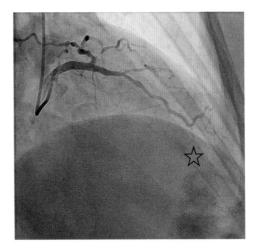

Figure 84.2

Contrast a large "wraparound LAD" that supplies the inferior wall of the LV (*left image; red star*) with that of a diminutive LAD, which terminates prior to the apex of the LV (*right image; blue star*).

PRESENTATION

A 53-year-old male with history of coronary artery disease (CAD; drug-eluting stent to right coronary artery [RCA] and left anterior descending coronary artery [LAD] approximately 1.5 years ago) is 8 days post-modified Whipple's procedure as part of pancreatic cancer management. While recovering in the hospital, he experienced a pulseless electrical activity arrest (PEA cardiac arrest).

Routine advanced life support (ACLS) was initiated and the patient had a return of spontaneous circulation. The following electrocardiogram (ECG) was obtained.

▶▶ **Presenting Electrocardiogram: Would You Activate the Cath Lab?**

ECG was obtained after the patient had return of spontaneous circulation.

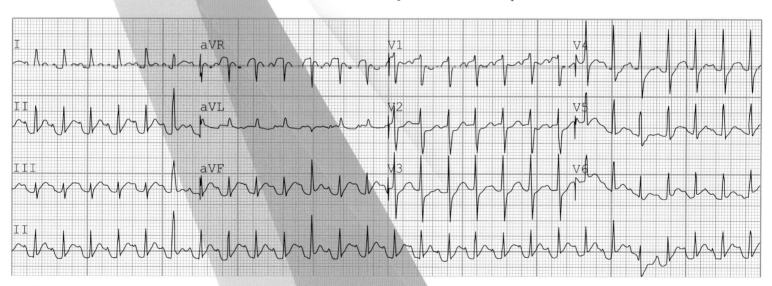

ECG 85.1

A prior ECG is available for comparison (see ECG 85.2).

▶▶ Prior Electrocardiogram for Comparison

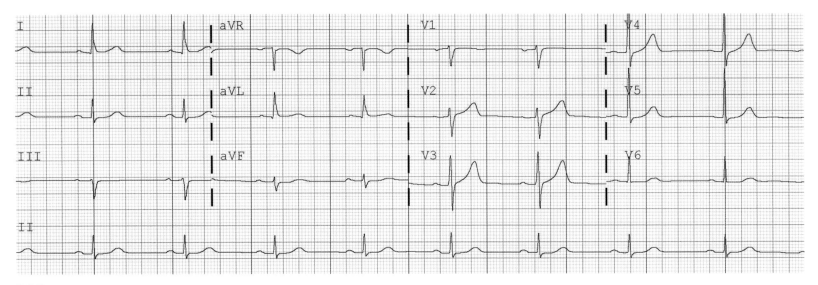

ECG 85.2

EXPLANATION

FEMI   The presenting ECG meets criteria for an inferior/posterior ST-segment elevation myocardial infarction (STEMI). However, this was not caused by an acute vessel closure.

It was revealed later by the primary surgical team that an intra-abdominal drain had been removed only a few minutes prior to the cardiac arrest. The patient had a PEA arrest due to an acute blood loss from intra-abdominal bleeding, which was discovered on autopsy. The serum hemoglobin had plummeted to 3.6 g/dL (*normal is 14 to 17 g/dL*).

It is important to not react to the first "major finding," which was the abnormal ECG post-cardiac arrest from PEA. The ST elevations were likely from acute anemia in addition to the consequences of cardiopulmonary resuscitation. Autopsy did not reveal an acute coronary syndrome as a contributor to the patient's death.

Case 86

PRESENTATION

A 74-year-old male with chronic tobacco use, hypertension, and dyslipidemia presents with ongoing low-grade intensity chest pain that started at rest.

There was no immediate action taken after the initial electrocardiogram (ECG), but when the serum troponin returned elevated at 1.8 ng/mL (normal range is <0.01 ng/mL), the cardiac catheterization team was activated.

▸▸ **Presenting Electrocardiogram: Would You Activate the Cath Lab?**

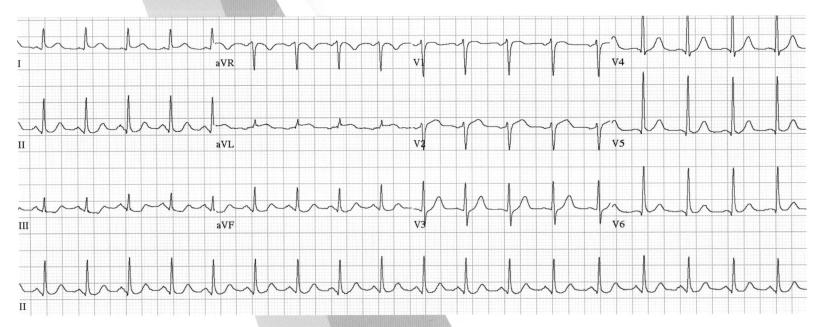

ECG 86.1

There is no prior ECG available for comparison.

EXPLANATION

FEMI   The presenting ECG demonstrates sinus tachycardia with ischemic-appearing ST depressions in the inferior leads, and submillimeter ST elevation in leads I and aVL. The elevations, however, do not meet ST-segment elevation myocardial infarction (STEMI) criteria.

Because the patient had persistent symptoms, abnormal ECG, and a mildly elevated troponin, he was referred for urgent angiography. The patient was found to have stable multivessel coronary artery disease (CAD) without a clear culprit lesion. There were high-grade lesions in the mid-left anterior descending coronary artery (LAD; with 70% stenosis), large left circumflex coronary artery (LCx)/OM$_2$ branch (with 80% stenosis), and mid-right coronary artery (RCA; with 70% stenosis). However, there was no plaque that appeared in newly ulcerated or blockages that could theoretically account for the acute lateral ST-segment changes. A left ventriculogram was performed, which demonstrated left ventricle (LV) wall motion abnormality consistent with an apical ballooning pattern of stress-induced cardiomyopathy. However, the coronary disease cannot explain the degree of wall motion abnormalities.

It is becoming recognized that underlying stable CAD (and in some instances, high-grade stable multivessel CAD as in this case) can coexist in patients presenting with stress-induced cardiomyopathy. In one study, 10% of patients who were found to have stress-induced cardiomyopathy have at least one vessel with >75% stenosis.[1]

It remains difficult to distinguish an acute coronary syndrome from an episode of this form of transient cardiomyopathy in an emergency department setting. Many clinical variables are often needed to help determine the correct diagnosis and occasionally a cardiac catheterization is required.[2]

This patient returned for an ECG and echocardiogram 3 months later, and the ST changes and LV function were normalized—all without coronary intervention or revascularization. This case also demonstrates the variable ECG presentation for cases of stress-induced cardiomyopathy. Review Cases 15, 22, and 60.

References

1. Kurisu S, Inoue I, Kawagoe T, et al. Prevalence of incidental coronary artery disease in Tako-tsubo cardiomyopathy. *Coron Artery Dis*. 2009;20(3):214-218.
2. Rawasia WF, Pachika A, Ikram S. Diagnostic dilemma: Takotsubo cardiomyopathy versus acute coronary syndrome. *J Invasive Cardiol*. 2014;26(6):E82-E84.

Case 87

PRESENTATION

A 63-year-old female with a history of a "thick heart" and paroxysmal atrial fibrilla-tion presents to the emergency department after suffering syncope in setting of a chronic recurrent chest pain episode. The patient remembers having a warm sensa-tion before finding herself waking up on the bathroom floor. She had regained full consciousness by the time she arrived to the emergency department.

She forgot to bring a copy of her baseline electrocardiogram (ECG) that her cardiologist gave her, but she had been told she has an "abnormal baseline ECG."

▸▸ **Presenting Electrocardiogram: Would You Activate the Cath Lab?**

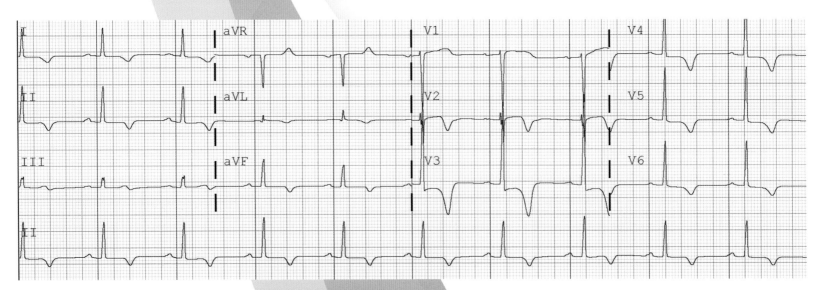

ECG 87.1

There is no prior ECG available for comparison.

EXPLANATION

FEMI The ECG demonstrates left ventricular hypertrophy (LVH) with deep T-wave inversions consistent with diffuse ischemia. Although there is 1-mm ST elevation in leads V_1 and V_2, the ECG does not meet criteria for an ST-segment elevation myocardial infarction (STEMI).

The ECG is a classic example of the findings of apical hypertrophic cardiomyopathy (Yamaguchi syndrome), which are LVH with deep symmetric T-wave inversions.[1]

The patient's syncope, after further history was obtained, seemed likely vasovagal in origin. She was kept for observation; serial ECG and troponins were unrevealing. Echocardiogram revealed a stable pattern of asymmetric LVH predominantly at the left ventricle (LV) apex.

Reference

1. Yamaguchi H, Ishimura T, Nishiyama S, et al. Hypertrophic nonobstructive cardiomyopathy with giant negative T waves (apical hypertrophy): ventriculographic and echocardiographic features in 30 patients. *Am J Cardiol.* 1979;44(3):401-412.

Case 88

PRESENTATION

A 72-year-old female with obesity, hypertension, and dyslipidemia presents from home after a witnessed cardiac arrest. Emergency personnel arrived at the scene and found the patient in ventricular fibrillation (VF). They were able to achieve return of spontaneous circulation before arriving to the emergency department.

▶▶ **Presenting Electrocardiogram: Would You Activate the Cath Lab?**

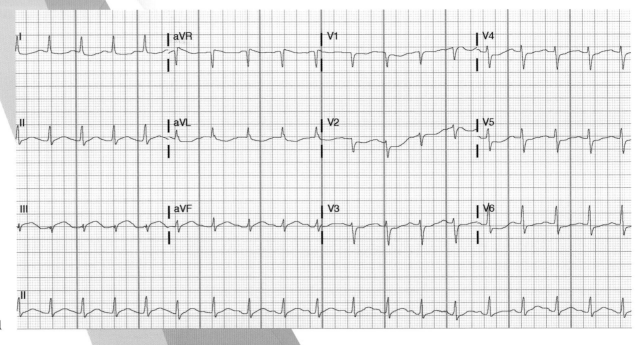

ECG 88.1

There is no prior electrocardiogram (ECG) available for comparison.

EXPLANATION

STEMI   The post-resuscitation ECG demonstrates sinus tachycardia with 1-mm ST elevations in III and aVF with horizontal ST depressions in leads V_2 to V_6 consistent with inferior–posterior infarction.

The patient had an acute left circumflex coronary artery (LCx)/OM_2 occlusion treated with angioplasty and stenting; her cardiac arrest from ventricular tachycardia (VT)/VF was undoubtedly secondary to the ST-segment elevation myocardial infarction (STEMI).

Underlying coronary artery disease (CAD) is present in most patients presenting with cardiac arrest; the presence of at least 1 significant coronary lesion is an exceedingly common finding in as high as 96% of cases of cardiac arrest due to VF and pulseless VT that presents with ST elevations on post-resuscitation ECG.[1] Among the predictors of survival includes successful angioplasty (others being not requiring inotropes on transport and a short time from cardiac arrest to successful return of spontaneous circulation).[2] This encourages us to consider coronary angiography in patients who survive cardiac arrest. Because of this, 2013 American College of Cardiology/American Heart Association (ACC/AHA) STEMI guidelines gave a Class I, Level of Evidence B recommendation for immediate angiography and percutaneous coronary intervention (PCI) for resuscitated out-of-hospital cardiac arrest patients whose initial ECG is consistent with STEMI.[3]

The management of post-VT/VF patients is not always so straightforward. There are both the diagnostic questions regarding the nature of the arrest and the management question regarding the risks and benefits of the procedure. For example:

1. Was the VT/VF cardiac arrest due to an acute coronary occlusion? Or was it a result of another pathologic process (ie, hypoxia from acute pulmonary disease, structural heart disease, medications/drugs, etc)?
2. What consideration should be given to the possibility of a limited meaningful neurologic recovery, especially when the time to first medical responder is prolonged?
3. Does the presenting ECG have ST elevations; what is the genesis of the ST abnormalities on ECG (ie, truly ischemic or from the metabolic derangements such as acidosis from the poor systemic perfusion caused by the arrest)?
4. What considerations should be given to the patient's baseline comorbidities, functional status, and bleeding risk, especially when they may not be known?
5. Is that patient stable enough to transfer from the emergency department to the cardiac catheterization laboratory?

The post-cardiac arrest ECG (when the patient is stable enough to obtain one) can be deceiving and can either demonstrate persistent ST elevation, transient ST elevation, or no ST elevations. **The presence of ST elevation in this setting does not necessarily indicate an acute infarction, and the absence of ST elevation does not mean absence of myocardial ischemia.** There is still a role for clinical judgment to determine if underlying ischemia is indeed the cause of the arrest. The nuances of ECG interpretation and the possible ECG outcomes of post-cardiac arrests are reviewed.

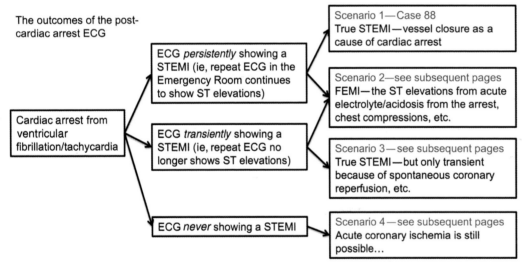

Figure 88.1

Scenario 2—Initial post-cardiac arrest ECG *transiently* demonstrating ST elevations but not due to coronary occlusion.

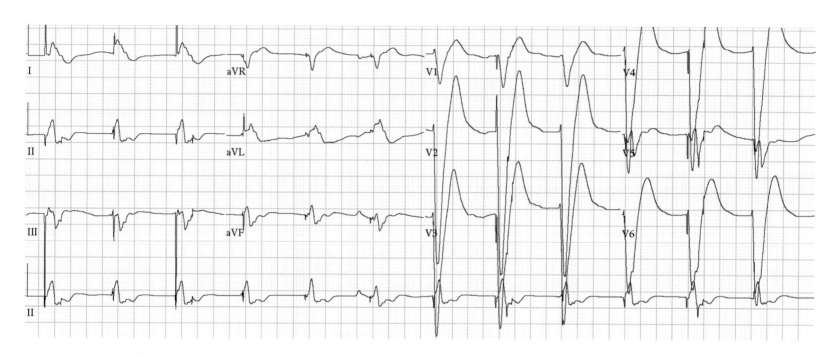

ECG 88.2

The ST elevations resolved after correction of acute electrolyte disturbances including hyperkalemia, acidosis, and hypoxia (ECG 88.2).

Scenario 3—Initial post-cardiac arrest ECG *transiently* demonstrating ST elevations, but with underlying unstable coronary lesion.

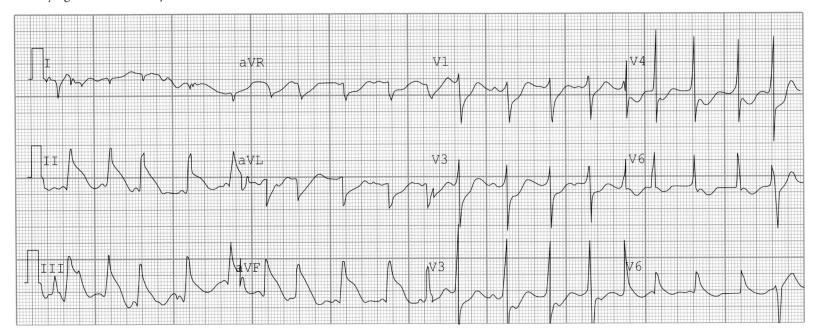

ECG 88.3a

ECG 88.3a was obtained after restoring spontaneous circulation of a patient with a witnessed cardiac arrest from VF. There is indeed inferior infarct pattern with posterior involvement. The inferior ST elevations resolved on arrival to the emergency department (see ECG 88.3b).

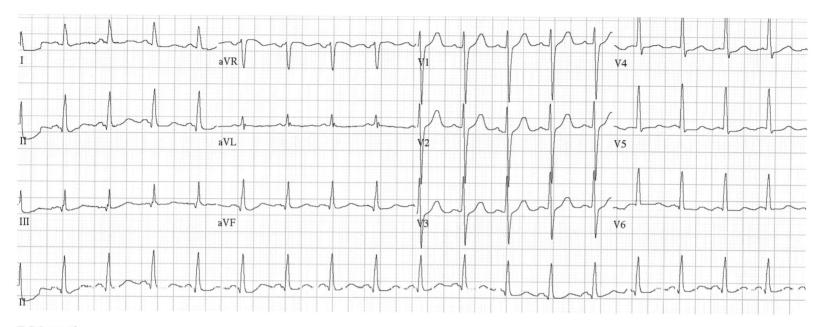

ECG 88.3b

ECG 88.3b shows resolution of the inferior ST elevations even prior to any coronary intervention.

It is possible for the ECG changes to resolve as a consequence of spontaneous coronary perfusion through naturally present anticoagulants or by medical therapy.[4] Review Case 80. Subsequent cardiac catheterization revealed an unstable proximal right coronary artery (RCA) lesion.

Scenario 4—Initial post-cardiac arrest *not* showing ST elevations.

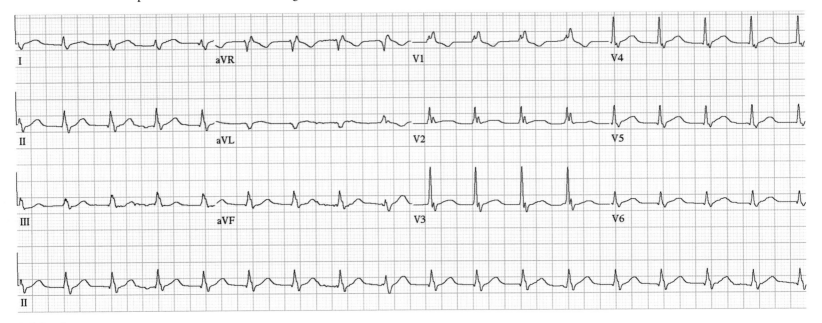

ECG 88.4

ECG 88.4 is of a 70-year-old patient who collapsed and was found to have VF. He was resuscitated in the field. His ECGs/rhythm strips never showed ST elevations; however, his left anterior descending coronary artery (LAD) was acutely thrombotic on emergent catheterization and undoubtedly the cause of the cardiac arrest.

References

1. Dumas F, Cariou A, Manzo-Silberman S, et al. Immediate percutaneous coronary intervention is associated with better survival after out-of-hospital cardiac arrest: insights from the PROCAT (Parisian Region Out of hospital Cardiac ArresT) registry. *Circ Cardiovasc Interv*. 2010;3(3):200-207.
2. Spaulding CM, Joly LM, Rosenberg A, et al. Immediate coronary angiography in survivors of out-of-hospital cardiac arrest. *N Engl J Med*. 1997;336(23):1629-1633.
3. O'Gara PT, Kushner FG, Ascheim DD et al. 2013 ACCF/AHA guideline for the management of ST-elevation myocardial infarction: executive summary: a report of the American College of Cardiology Foundation/American Heart Association Task Force on Practice Guidelines. *J Am Coll Cardiol*. 2013;61(4):485-510.
4. Bainey KR, Fu Y, Wagner GS, et al.; ASSENT 4 PCI Investigators. Spontaneous reperfusion in ST-elevation myocardial infarction: comparison of angiographic and electrocardiographic assessments. *Am Heart J*. 2008;156(2):248-255.

Case 89

PRESENTATION

A 45-year-old female with mental retardation from a group home presents with altered mental status. In the emergency department, she was intubated for airway protection and had developed pulseless electrical activity (PEA) cardiac arrest.

The patient was noted to be hypothermic with rectal temperature under 30°C. An electrocardiogram (ECG) was obtained.

▶▶ **Presenting Electrocardiogram: Would You Activate the Cath Lab?**

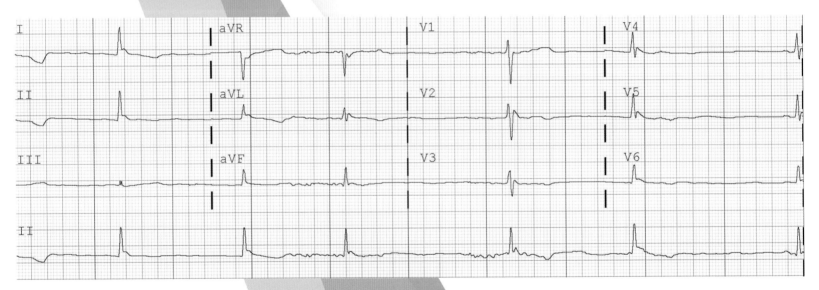

ECG 89.1

There is no prior ECG available for comparison.

EXPLANATION

FEMI   The presenting ECG demonstrates atrial fibrillation with slow ventricular response, intraventricular conduction delay, and prolonged QT. There is indeed J-point elevation at the ST segment. This is most consistent with an Osborn wave of severe hypothermia.

It is believed that hypothermia affects the normal voltage gradient between the ventricular epicardial and endocardial layers, and results in the noticeable J wave.[1] The presenting ECG does not meet criteria for ST-segment elevation myocardial infarction (STEMI) nor is it suggestive of ischemia. With re-warming, the ST-segment changes resolved (see ECG 89.3).

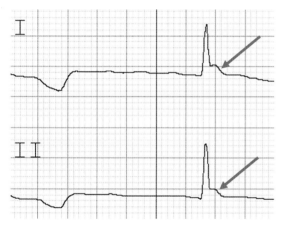

ECG 89.2

Blue arrows point to the Osborn waves.

ECG 89.3

ECG 89.3 was obtained after rewarming the patient. The patient's rhythm reverted to sinus rhythm from atrial fibrillation, and there is resolution of the Osborn waves.

Reference

1. Yan GX, Antzelevitch C. Cellular basis for the electrocardiographic J wave. *Circulation*. 1996;93(2):372-379.

Case 90

PRESENTATION

A 79-year-old man presents complaining of not feeling well for the past 5 days. He has a history of nonischemic cardiomyopathy, biventricular automated implantable cardioverter defibrillator (AICD), and a previous history of ventricular tachycardia (VT) with prior VT ablation. He has been taken off amiodarone due to concerns of amiodarone-induced pulmonary toxicity.

He presents to his physician for nonspecific progressive fatigue. An electrocardiogram (ECG) was obtained.

▶▶ **Presenting Electrocardiogram: Would You Activate the Cath Lab?**

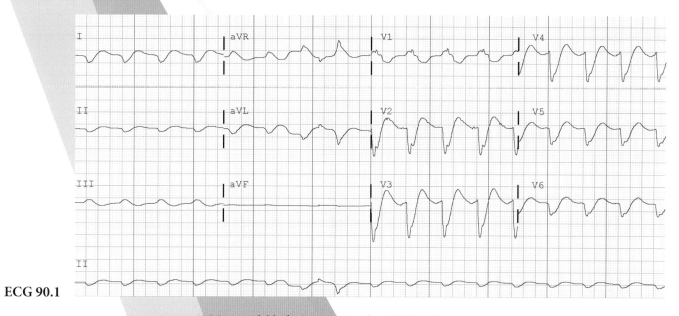

ECG 90.1

A prior ECG is available for comparison (see ECG 90.2).

▶▶ Prior Electrocardiogram for Comparison

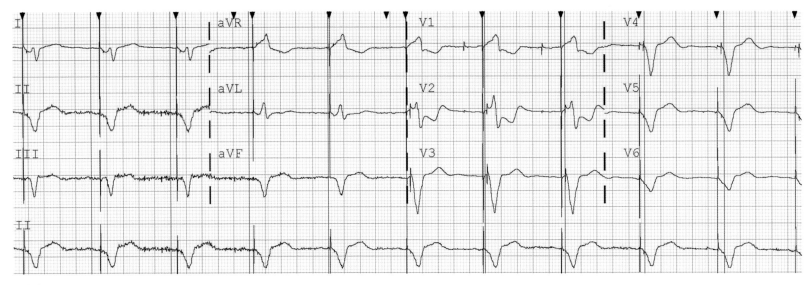

ECG 90.2

EXPLANATION

FEMI   The key here is to recognize that the ECG demonstrates slow VT. The baseline ECG shows normal biventricular pacing. At a quick glance, the ST segment appears very abnormal and can easily be mistaken for an ischemic episode.

Given the patient's history of VT and recent medication changes, recurrent scar-mediated monomorphic VT was likely. Note episodes of **polymorphic** VT may have a stronger correlation with acute myocardial ischemia. The recognition of VT starts by noting the marked prolonged QRS interval, which in this case is approximately 200 ms. Several algorithms have been studied to help determine the presence of VT (usually in context of differentiating VT vs supraventricular tachycardia with aberrancy). Among these include the Brugada algorithm and an 1-lead aVR method; in-depth discussion on this matter is beyond the scope of this book.[1,2] However, ECG findings that indicate VT on the presenting ECG includes the prolonged QRS duration, monophasic R in V_1 despite having a right bundle branch block (RBBB) morphology, and initial R wave in aVR.

The patient was referred for another VT ablation procedure.

References

1. Brugada P, Brugada J, Mont L, et al. A new approach to the differential diagnosis of a regular tachycardia with a wide QRS complex. *Circulation*. 1991;83(5):1649-1659.
2. Vereckei A, Duray G, Szenasi G, et al. Application of a new algorithm in the differential diagnosis of wide QRS complex tachycardia. *Eur Heart J*. 2007;28(5):589-600.

Case 91

PRESENTATION

A 52-year-old male with lifelong tobacco use and active "abdominal cancer" was brought into the emergency department by his girlfriend because of aphasia and complete right-sided weakness of 3 days duration. There was no chest pain or shortness of breath reported.

As part of the evaluation of stroke in the emergency department, an electrocardiogram (ECG) was performed. Aside from hypertension, all other vital signs were stable.

▶▶ **Presenting Electrocardiogram: Would You Activate the Cath Lab?**

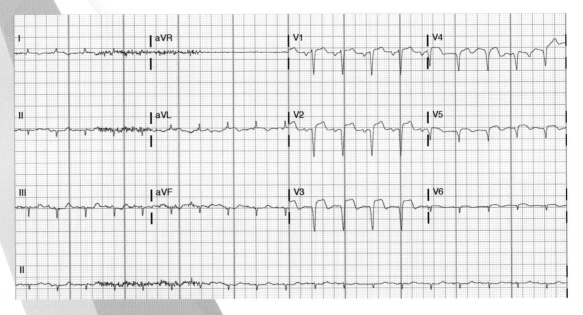

ECG 91.1

A prior ECG is available for comparison (see ECG 91.2).

▶▶ Prior Electrocardiogram for Comparison

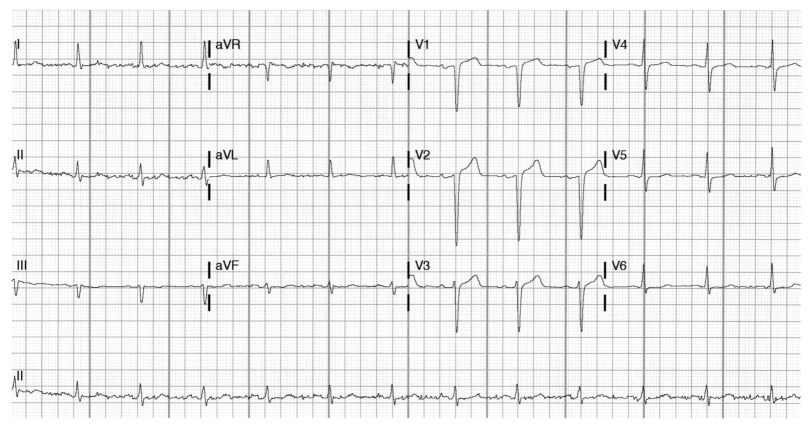

ECG 91.2

EXPLANATION

 STEMI   The presenting ECG demonstrates age-indeterminate extensive anteroseptal and anterior myocardial infarction.

However, the next major clinical decision was whether an emergent cardiac catheterization would be safe/beneficial in setting of a concomitant massive subacute stroke as well as active underlying malignancy, which turned out to be stage 4 widely metastatic renal cell carcinoma. The patient did not present with chest pain symptoms and the ECG had already demonstrated extensive anteroseptal/anterior Q waves, which implies a completed infarction.

There is a substantial risk for intracranial hemorrhage conversion in this patient who had recently suffered a large right middle cerebral artery (MCA) infarction, especially when full dose antithrombotic medications are administered for purposes of coronary intervention. In fact, an acute stroke is considered a "relative contraindication" for coronary angiography.[1]

Furthermore, the patient was stable from a cardiac standpoint, without evidence of hemodynamic instability or arrhythmias. Finally, this patient has widely metastatic malignancy, which is a "severe concomitant illness that drastically shortens life expectancy"—another key aspect in determining the appropriateness of pursuing an urgent cardiac procedure.[1]

On echocardiogram the next morning, a left ventricular thrombus was noted, which was likely the result of an asymptomatic large left anterior descending coronary artery (LAD) occlusion. Cerebral embolization likely caused the patient's stroke. **If a catheterization had been performed in the emergent setting without knowledge of the left ventricle (LV) thrombus, crossing the aortic valve with a catheter for standard LV pressure measurement and left ventriculogram could have led to additional systemic embolization.**

Acting on the new abnormal ECG may have perhaps been the reflexive choice, as the cardiac issue can be perceived as more "treatable" compared to his advanced malignancy and the subacute stroke. However, this may have resulted in more harm than benefit. The patient ultimately decided for hospice as he never recovered from the debilitating stroke with underlying incurable malignancy (Figures 91.1 and 91.2).

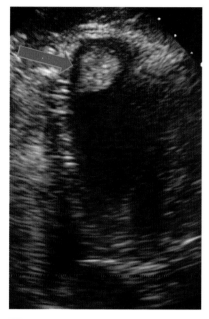

Figure 91.1

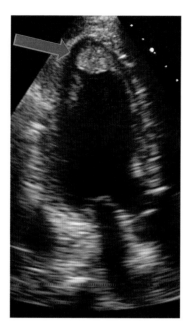

Figure 91.2

The patient in this case had a large LV thrombus as demonstrated on echocardiogram (*red arrow*). The genesis of the LV thrombus was likely from the recent asymptomatic LAD occlusion, which led to blood stasis in the apical LV and potentially myocardial edema/inflammation, which can be a nidus for the thrombus formation. Pieces of the freshly formed LV thrombus likely then embolized into the brain and caused the massive stroke.

Reference

1. Scanlon PJ, Faxon DP, Audet AM, et al. ACC/AHA guidelines for coronary angiography. A report of the American College of Cardiology/American Heart Association Task Force on practice guidelines (Committee on Coronary Angiography). Developed in collaboration with the Society for Cardiac Angiography and Interventions. *J Am Coll Cardiol.* 1999;33(6):1756-1824.

Case 92

PRESENTATION

A 46-year-old male with history of aortic valve endocarditis presents with profound heart failure symptoms from severe aortic insufficiency. After stabilization, he had a successful mechanical aortic valve replacement. Prior to his valve surgery, he had a cardiac catheterization that revealed normal coronaries.

On postoperative day 7, the surgical team obtained a routine electrocardiogram (ECG) and noted progressive ST changes, despite improving clinically. The patient denied any chest pain.

▶▶ **Presenting Electrocardiogram: Would You Activate the Cath Lab?**

ECG performed 7 days after valve replacement surgery.

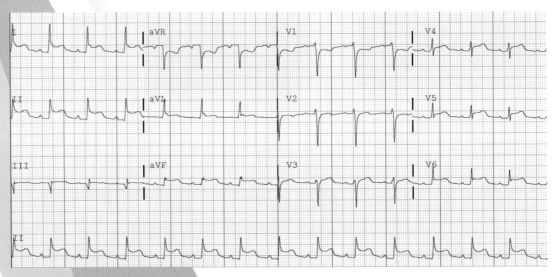

ECG 92.1

A prior ECG from immediately after valve surgery is available for comparison (see ECG 92.2).

▶▶ Prior Electrocardiogram for Comparison

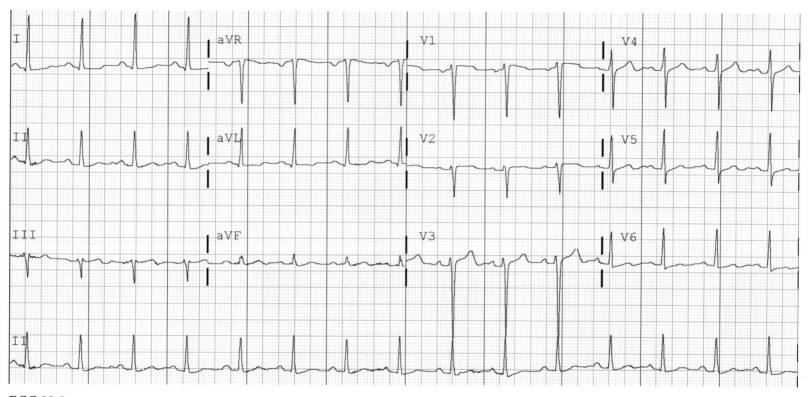

ECG 92.2

EXPLANATION

 FEMI   The ECG demonstrates inferior and lateral ST elevations, which independently would be concerning for acute myocardial infarction.

ECGs obtained post–open heart surgery may demonstrate ST changes. These findings postoperatively may be as a consequence of the hemodynamic changes, myocardial injury from surgical technique, and disruption of the pericardium. Evaluation of these ECG changes in the postoperative patient, to determine the presence an acute coronary syndrome, must incorporate both the clinical presentation and the patient's appropriateness for cardiac catheterization during the postoperative recovery phase.

This patient's echocardiogram revealed a small-to-moderate pericardial effusion with normal wall motions. With these reassuring noninvasive findings, given the patient's overall benign recovery and lack of chest pain symptoms, the diagnosis was made of postoperative pericarditis. The patient did not need a cardiac catheterization.

Echocardiogram of the patient demonstrated small-to-moderate pericardial effusion (*noted by the blue arrows*). The ST elevations were likely a result of postoperative pericarditis with associated pericardial effusion (Figures 92.1 and 92.2).

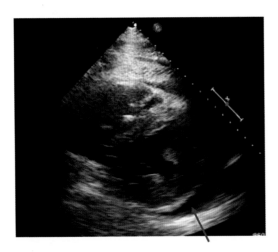

Figure 92.1

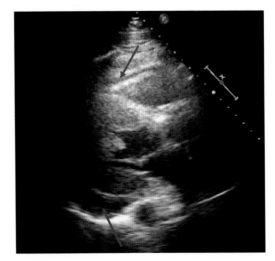

Figure 92.2

Case 93

PRESENTATION

A 65-year-old male with gastroesophageal reflux disease (GERD) presents with worsening dyspnea for the past month. He notes his exercise capacity has greatly diminished over the past couple weeks. There is a vague component of chest pain, which he describes as resembling "heartburn."

In the emergency department, his vitals were notable for a blood pressure of 130/80, heart rate of 89 bpm, and oxygenation was in the mid-90%.

▸▸ **Presenting Electrocardiogram: Would You Activate the Cath Lab?**

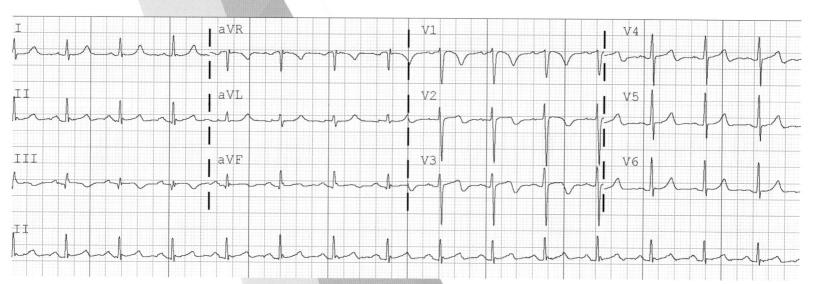

ECG 93.1

A prior electrocardiogram (ECG) is available for comparison (see ECG 93.2).

▶▶ Prior Electrocardiogram for Comparison

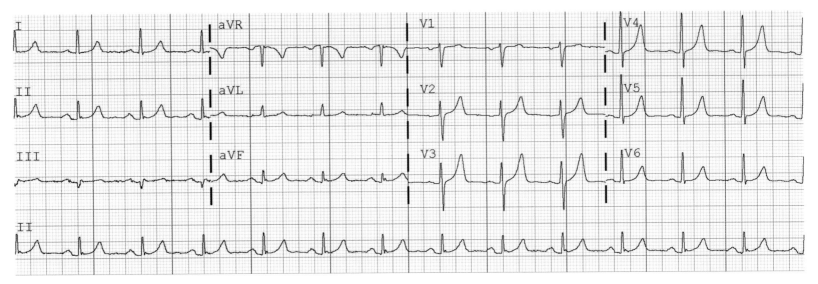

ECG 93.2

EXPLANATION

FEMI   The presenting ECG meets borderline ST-segment elevation myocardial infarction (STEMI) criteria, with 1-mm elevation in V_2 and V_3 and new biphasic anterior T waves.

The key to this case is to appreciate that these new ST changes were not from acute coronary disease, but rather from sub-massive pulmonary embolism. An urgent cardiac catheterization was performed; however, it was unrevealing for high-grade coronary artery disease (CAD) or left ventricle (LV) dysfunction. Because of substantial ECG changes (along with serum troponins which eventually returned as positive), a computed tomography (CT) scan to rule out pulmonary embolism was ordered. It revealed large bilateral pulmonary artery emboli extending into multiple lobar and segmental branches with evidence of right ventricle (RV) enlargement.

Sub-massive or massive pulmonary embolism is associated with ECG changes including sinus tachycardia, S1Q3T3, right bundle branch block (RBBB), and anterior T-wave inversions that may appear "Wellens'-like." These changes are thought to reflect a degree of acute right heart strain associated with a large burden of pulmonary embolus. This case showcases pulmonary embolism as an important differential diagnosis in patients who presents with chest symptoms and an abnormal ECG. Review Case 68.

Filling defects (*blue arrows*) in the bilateral pulmonary arteries indicating pulmonary embolism (Figure 93.1). Right heart strain noted—this likely contributed to abnormal ECG findings (Figure 93.2). Note the right ventricular (*red star*) size is greater than the left ventricular (*blue star*) size.

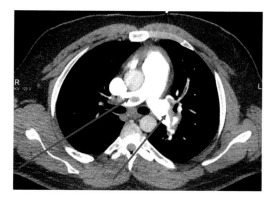

Figure 93.1

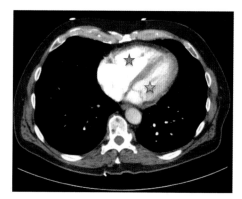

Figure 93.2

Case 94

PRESENTATION

A 28-year-old morbidly obese male with asthma presents with 2 days of worsening shortness of breath and increasing substernal chest pain.

His blood pressure was 135/88, heart rate 103 bpm, and his saturation was 99% on room air.

▸▸ **Presenting Electrocardiogram: Would You Activate the Cath Lab?**

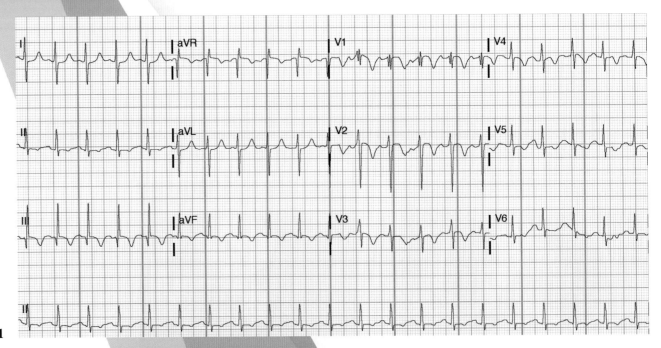

ECG 94.1

There is no prior electrocardiogram (ECG) available for comparison.

EXPLANATION

FEMI   Although there was 1-mm ST in lead V_1 and 2-mm ST in lead V_2, along with biphasic T waves in the anterior (Wellens'-like) and inferior leads, this was a case of bilateral massive pulmonary embolism. Note the sinus tachycardia and the S1Q3T3 pattern.

The patient had right ventricular dysfunction/strain noted on both the subsequent computed tomography (CT) scan and echocardiogram—which was the likely cause of the ECG ST-T abnormalities. The cardiac catheterization was appropriately canceled in this case by the interventional cardiologist. This patient eventually required emergent intravenous (IV) tissue plasminogen activator (tPA) therapy.

Remember that anterior ST changes (including mild anterior ST elevations, and "Wellens'-like" changes) may reflect acute right ventricle (RV) strain of massive pulmonary embolism, and not necessarily an acute coronary syndrome. Review Cases 68 and 93.

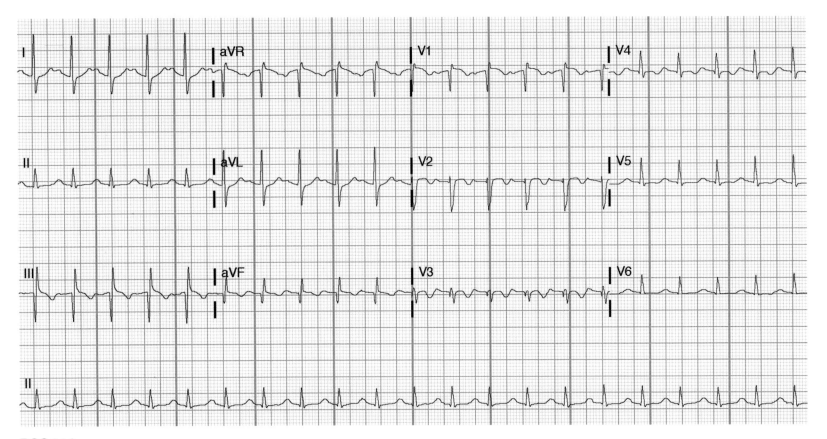

ECG 94.2

ECG 94.2 is another example of a patient with massive pulmonary embolism who had new is-chemic appearing ST changes on ECG.

Case 95

PRESENTATION

An 86-year-old male with a dual chamber pacemaker presents to an orthopedic clinic with left knee pain and swelling. An arthrocentesis was performed in the procedure room.

A routine electrocardiogram (ECG) was obtained per protocol and because it was "abnormal," the patient was directed to the emergency department. The patient denies chest pain or shortness of breath.

▶▶ **Presenting Electrocardiogram: Would You Activate the Cath Lab?**

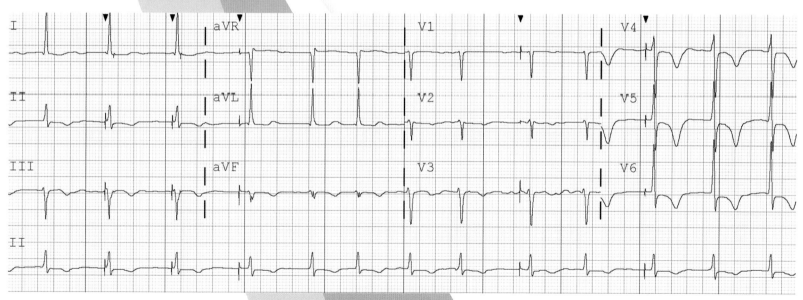

ECG 95.1

A repeat ECG was performed (see ECG 95.2).

▶▶ Repeat Electrocardiogram: Would You Activate the Cath Lab?

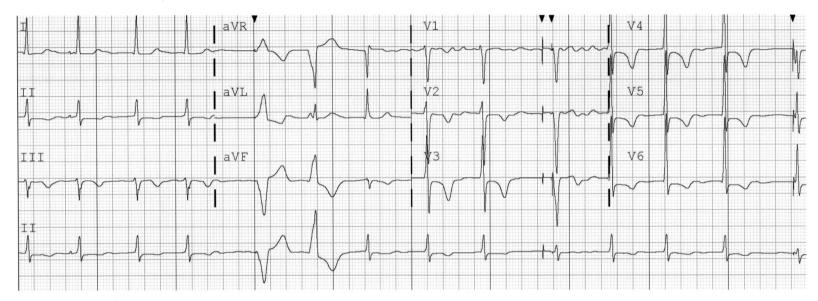

ECG 95.2

Another repeat ECG was performed (see ECG 95.3).

▶▶ **Repeat Electrocardiogram: Would You Activate the Cath Lab?**

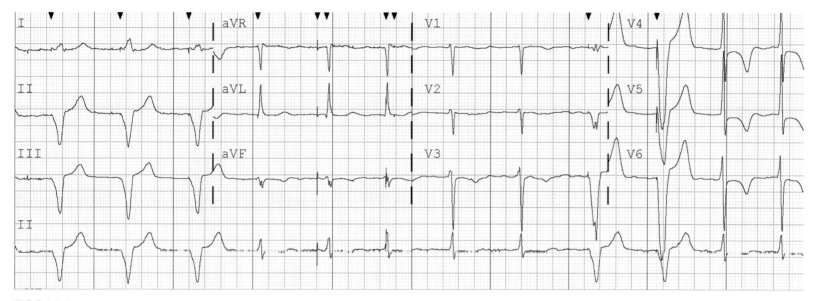

ECG 95.3

A prior ECG is available for comparison (see ECG 95.4).

▶▶ Prior Electrocardiogram for Comparison

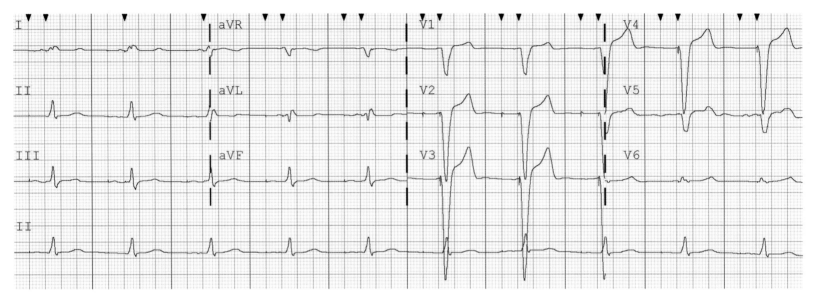

ECG 95.4

EXPLANATION

FEMI   The ECG demonstrates atrial fibrillation and diffuse T-wave inversions suspicious for global ischemia. There are ventricular pacing spikes without capture because of native ventricular conduction. Notably, on the beats, the patient is not receiving ventricular pacing; the T waves are inverted.

The deep anterior and lateral T-wave inversion on the non-paced beats (better seen on the repeat ECG) are an example of **"T-wave memory"** or **Cardiac Memory**. This is a benign finding and likely represents a non-clinically important modification in repolarization channels after a period of abnormal depolarization/repolarization, such as with cardiac pacing. This can also be seen as a result of intermittent left bundle branch block (LBBB), frequent premature ventricular contractions (PVCs), or conduction down a bypass track (as in Wolff–Parkinson–White syndrome). Cardiac memory can arise within minutes of pacing and its resolution on ECG may depend on the duration of pacing.[1]

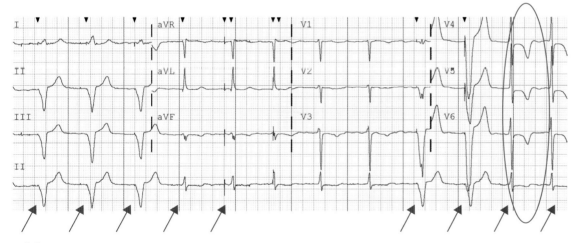

ECG 95.5

In review of the rhythm strip in lead II, compare the T waves while ventricular-paced (*blue arrows*) with the T waves when not-ventricular-paced (*red arrows*). The marked T-wave inversions, which are most prominent on leads V_4 to V_6 (*red circle*), are a manifestation of T-wave memory and not myocardial ischemia.

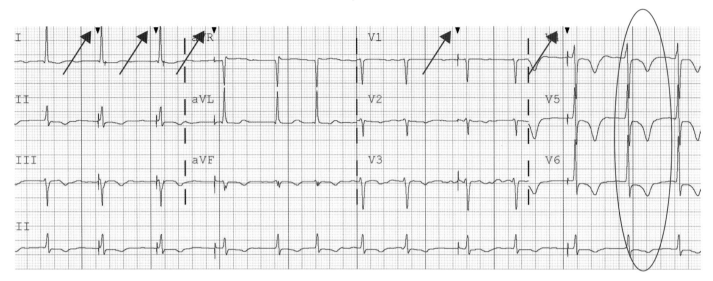

ECG 95.6

Review the presenting ECG. Although it may appear the patient had intermittent ventricular pacing spikes with the ECG-machine labeling each pacer spike (*blue arrow*), the heart actually did not "require" the ventricular pacing and had full underlying native conduction on this ECG. Note the T-wave inversions of T-wave memory (*red circle*) that is best noted on the lateral V₄ to V₆ leads.

Reference

1. Shvilkin A, Huang HD, Josephson ME. Cardiac memory: diagnostic tool in the making. *Circ Arrhythm Electrophysiol.* 2015;8(2):475-482.

Case 96

PRESENTATION

A 70-year-old female with history of congestive heart failure with normal left ventricle (LV) function was diagnosed with ischemic colitis that required right hemicolectomy. Her recovery was complicated by septic shock. Two weeks post-operation, the patient complains of acute onset chest heaviness with difficulty breathing. The initial troponin T was minimally detected at 0.03 ng/mL (normal range is <0.01 ng/mL) but the electrocardiogram (ECG) was abnormal.

▶▶ **Presenting Electrocardiogram: Would You Activate the Cath Lab?**

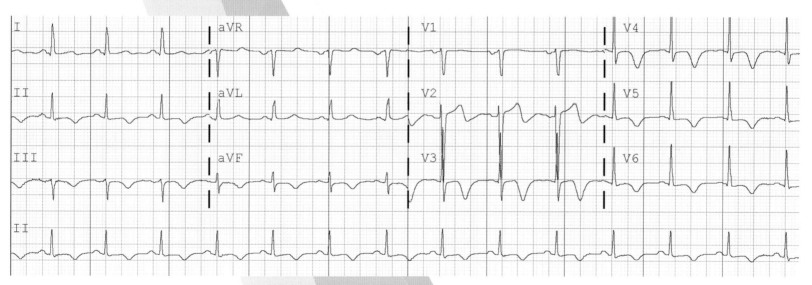

ECG 96.1

A prior ECG is available for comparison (see ECG 96.2).

▶▶ Prior Electrocardiogram for Comparison

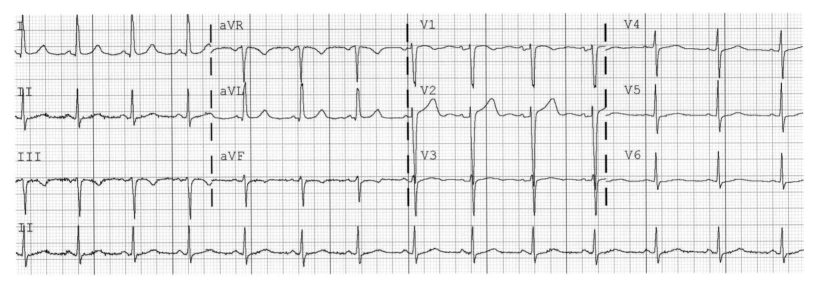

ECG 96.2

EXPLANATION

FEMI   Despite significant ST-T changes resembling ischemia with a prominent "Wellens' T-wave" appearance, coronary angiogram revealed no acute coronary lesions.

Ventriculogram revealed wall motion abnormalities consistent with a stress-induced cardiomyopathy. In this setting, coronary angiography remains the best way to exclude acute coronary artery disease (CAD) as a cause of the marked ECG changes.

Review Cases 22, 60, and 86.

Case 97

PRESENTATION

The same patient from Case 96 returns to the hospital 1.5 years later with acute nausea and vomiting consistent with gastroenteritis. She had severe hypotension from hypovolemia. She was admitted to the medical intensive care unit.

The patient reports of dyspnea and new chest discomfort, which she admits may be from her underlying panic disorder.

An electrocardiogram (ECG) was obtained.

▸▸ **Presenting Electrocardiogram: Would You Activate the Cath Lab?**

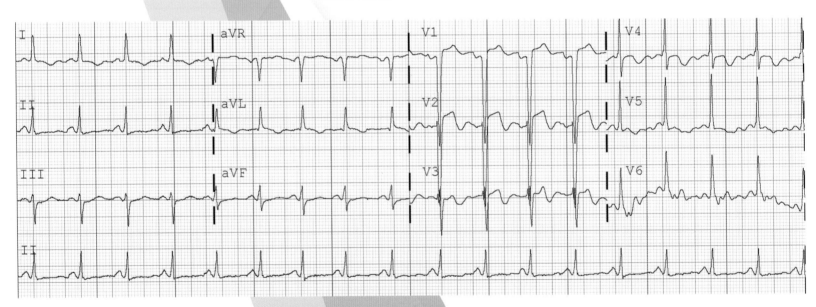

ECG 97.1

A prior ECG (after the patient recovered from her stress-induced cardiomyopathy 1.5 years ago) is available for comparison (see ECG 97.2).

▶▶ Prior Electrocardiogram for Comparison

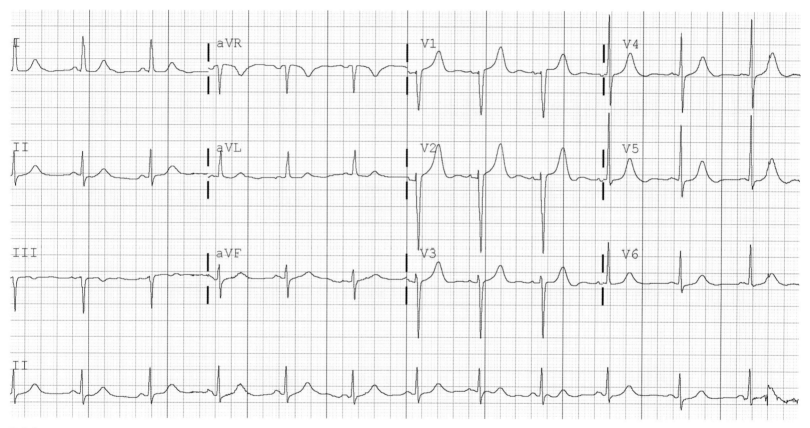

ECG 97.2

EXPLANATION

 FEMI   The initial ECG demonstrates sinus tachycardia, left ventricular hypertrophy (LVH), with new anteroseptal/anterior ST elevations consistent with infarction.

The patient was referred for another urgent coronary angiogram. Angiography did reveal a 100% stenosis of a small distal left circumflex coronary artery (LCx) vessel but with the distal LCx supplied by left-to-left collaterals; there was nonobstructive coronary artery disease (CAD) in the other vessels. Echocardiogram and left ventriculogram revealed severely reduced ejection fraction with left ventricle (LV) apical ballooning. The new angiogram findings in the distal LCx lesion (which was not present on the angiogram 1.5 years ago) do not explain the ECG findings (anterior ST-T changes) or the apical LV wall motion abnormalities. In light of the severe gastroenteritis, a case of **recurrent stress-induced cardiomyopathy** was diagnosed. Medical therapy was recommended and the patient's cardiomyopathy recovered in subsequent follow-up evaluation.

Stress-induced cardiomyopathy is believed to involve catecholamine surge and the awareness of this syndrome has increased since its initial description in 1991.

Recurrence of this syndrome is believed to occur in approximately 5% of patients.[1] High-grade CAD, which is not the cause of this transient LV dysfunction, can be seen in patients with stress-induced cardiomyopathy.[2] Review Case 86.

References

1. Singh K, Carson K, Usmani Z, Sawhney G, Shah R, Horowitz J. Systematic review and meta-analysis of incidence and correlates of recurrence of Takotsubo cardiomyopathy. *Int J Cardiol.* 2014;174(3):696-701.
2. Kurisu S, Inoue I, Kawagoe T, et al. Prevalence of incidental coronary artery disease in Tako-tsubo cardiomyopathy. *Coron Artery Dis.* 2009;20(3):214-218.

Case 98

PRESENTATION

A 72-year-old male with previous left anterior descending coronary artery (LAD) stent presents with acute left forearm pain with exertion.

▶▶ **Presenting Electrocardiogram: Would You Activate the Cath Lab?**

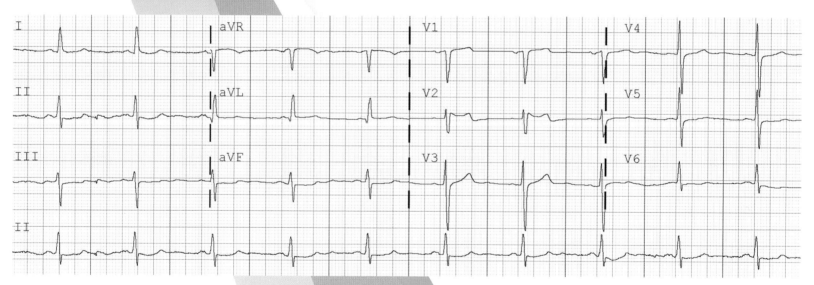

ECG 98.1

A prior electrocardiogram (ECG) is available for comparison (see ECG 98.2).

▶▶ Prior Electrocardiogram for Comparison

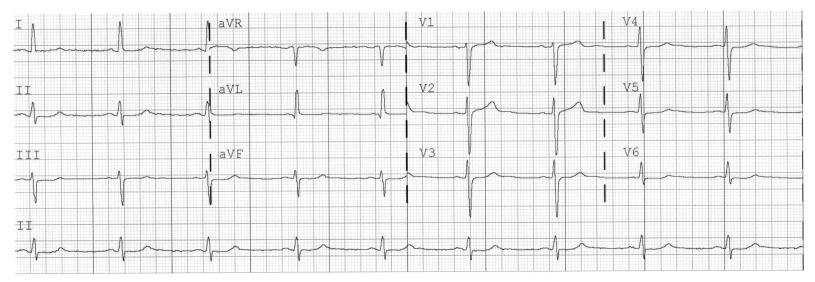

ECG 98.2

EXPLANATION

FEMI   There is ST elevation in V_2 that appeared suspicious for ischemia, but it was only in 1 lead without any abnormalities in the contiguous leads. This is not diagnostic of coronary ischemia.

With the patient's presenting anginal-like symptoms, new abnormal ECG findings, and previous cardiac history, the clinical suspicion was high enough to perform coronary angiography. Urgent cardiac catheterization showed a patent LAD stent, with mild/moderate stenosis in other vessels.

In retrospect, the new abnormal ST-T contours in lead V_2 could potentially be from lead placement, or even possibly a transient Brugada-like "saddle-back" pattern (Type 2); review Case 73.

A repeat ECG that was performed after the cardiac catheterization demonstrated the patient's baseline ST-segment contours with resolution of the ST changes in lead V_2. Serum troponins were negative.

Case 99

A 38-year-old male with sickle cell disease without known cardiac issues presents with acute onset left-sided substernal chest pressure with a squeezing quality.

▸▸ **Presenting Electrocardiogram: Would You Activate the Cath Lab?**

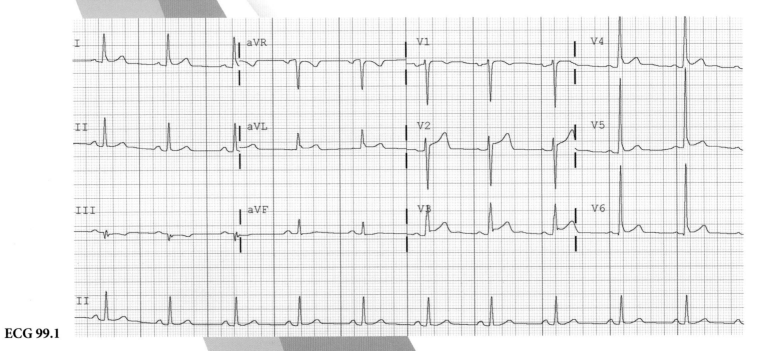

ECG 99.1

There is no prior electrocardiogram (ECG) available for comparison.

EXPLANATION

FEMI The ECG shows left ventricular hypertrophy coronary artery (LVH) with anterior ST elevations, which are indeed concerning for anterior ischemia.

However, cardiac catheterization revealed no coronary artery disease with normal left ventricular (LV) function. Overall, the ST-segment changes are consistent with ECG pattern of early repolarization. Review Case 10.

The ST-segment elevation can be described as "J-point elevation without end QRS notching/slurring"—leads V_2 and V_3; and "QRS slurring with ST elevation"—leads V_4 to V_6, and aVL. Recognizing these patterns can be helpful to distinguish true ST-segment elevation myocardial infarction (STEMI) from its mimics.

The patient was diagnosed with acute chest syndrome from his sickle cell disease.

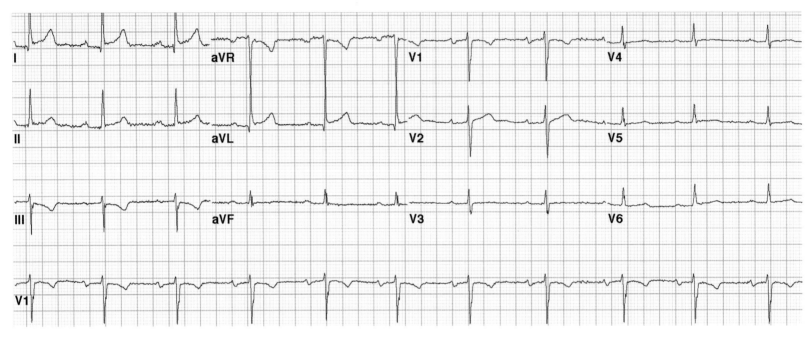

ECG 99.2

ECG 99.2 depicts another example of early repolarization in a patient who presented for evaluation of atypical chest pain. Note the ST elevations in leads I and aVL, which may be concerning for an isolated high-lateral myocardial infarction (MI). Without a previous ECG to compare to, the decision to pursue urgent catheterization relies heavily on clinical judgment. The concave nature of the ST segment ("smiley face" orientation) and atypical symptoms were key findings in avoiding an urgent catheterization in this case.

Case 100

PRESENTATION

A 54-year-old female with lifelong tobacco and significant alcohol abuse was found after a syncopal episode near her car. Initially, she had no complaints, but she started to develop substernal chest pain while she was in the hospital. Serial troponin Ts were increasing, from 0.3 ng/dL → 2.5 ng/mL → 3.8 ng/mL (normal range is <0.01 ng/mL).

Electrocardiograms (ECGs) were performed.

▸▸ **Presenting Electrocardiogram: Would You Activate the Cath Lab?**

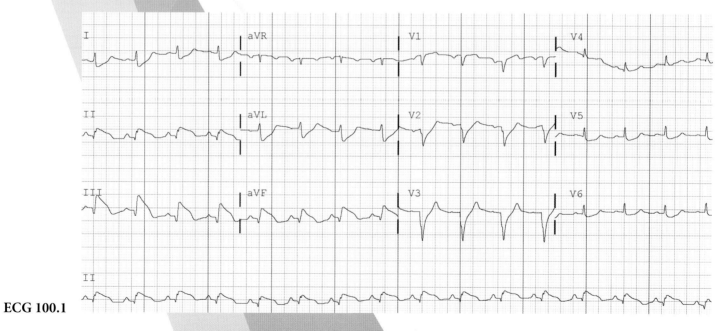

ECG 100.1

A prior ECG is available for comparison (see ECG 100.2).

▶▶ Prior Electrocardiogram for Comparison

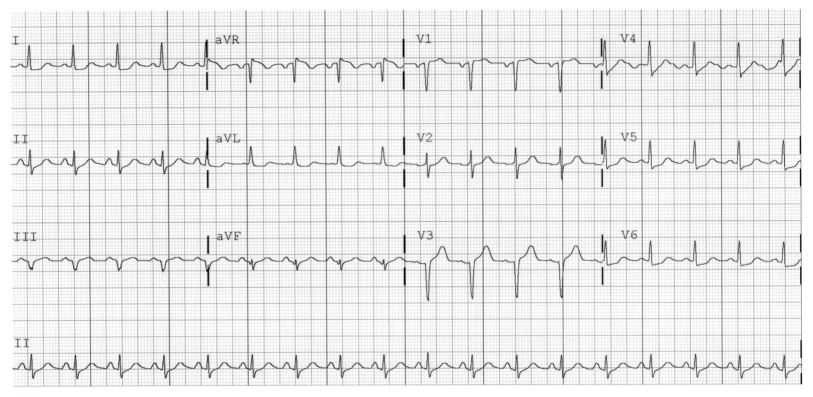

ECG 100.2

EXPLANATION

 STEMI   The ECG shows true inferior ST elevation, with diffuse ST depressions consistent with global ischemia.

Cardiac catheterization would reveal that there was indeed coronary occlusion, but not from thrombus or plaque—rather, there was dramatic severe triple-vessel coronary spasm. Injection of intracoronary nitroglycerin relieved the spasm in all 3 major epicardial vessels with complete resolution of the ECG changes.

Her urine drug screen returned positive for urine amphetamines. Precipitants of coronary artery spasm include stimulants (ie, amphetamines), cocaine, severe cold, severe physical/emotional stress, severe hypomagnesemia (not exhibited by the patient), and alcohol consumption. Note that patients with underlying coronary artery disease (CAD), and therefore a degree of endothelial dysfunction, have a higher likelihood to develop coronary artery spasm.[1]

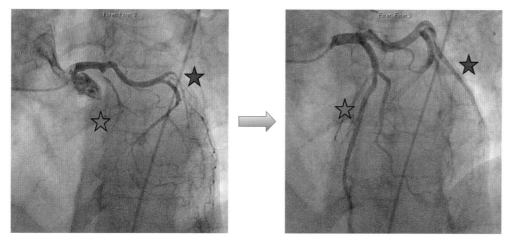

Figure 100.1   **Figure 100.2**

Resolution of coronary spasm can be seen in the right-hand image in both the left anterior descending coronary artery (LAD; *blue star*) and the left circumflex coronary artery (LCx; *red star*) after injection of intracoronary nitroglycerin.

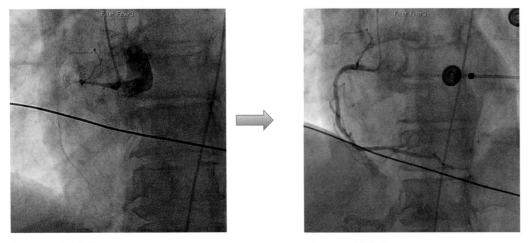

Figure 100.3   Figure 100.4

Resolution of coronary spasm can be seen in the right-hand image in the right coronary artery (RCA) after injection of intracoronary nitroglycerin.

Reference

1. Hung MJ, Hu P, Hung MY. Coronary artery spasm: review and update. *Int J Med Sci.* 2014;11(11):1161-1171.

Index

Note: Page numbers followed by "*f*" refer to figures.